AI in Mental Health Nursing

Digital Tools, Clinical Decision Support, Ethics, and Practical Integration Strategies for Psychiatric Nurses and Mental Health Professionals

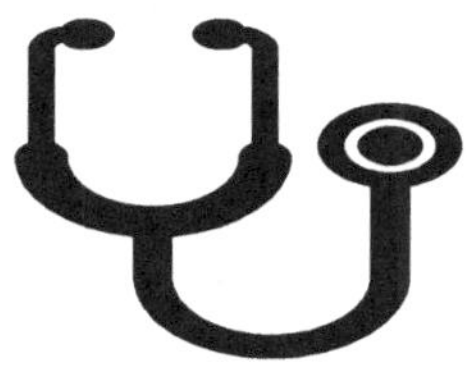

How Mental Health Nurses Can Harness AI Tools, Reduce Burnout, and Deliver Evidence-Based Digital Care

Conor Gino Pettersson

First Edition, November, 2025

ISBN: 978-1-923646-14-8

Table of Contents

Why Every Mental Health Nurse Needs to Be AI-Ready

You probably don't realize it, but AI is already part of your workday. Maybe you've noticed the new risk assessment tool that flags patients differently than you expected. Perhaps your trust implemented a digital triage system last quarter. Or maybe you've seen colleagues using voice-to-text documentation software that somehow knows medical terminology better than your phone's autocorrect.

Here's what's happening: **artificial intelligence** has moved from the realm of science fiction into the daily operations of mental health services across the UK. While you were managing caseloads and documenting care plans, AI quietly embedded itself in NHS systems. The question isn't whether you'll work with AI—you already are. The question is whether you'll understand what's happening well enough to use these tools effectively and advocate for your patients when the algorithms get it wrong.

The Reality Check: AI Is Already in Your Trust

Let me be direct. If you work in mental health nursing in 2025, you're interacting with AI systems whether you know it or not. NHS England has invested millions in digital transformation initiatives, and AI tools are being deployed across trusts at an accelerating pace (NHS England, 2023).

Limbic Access, an AI-powered triage system, is now active in over 100 NHS talking therapy services, handling more than 200,000 referrals (Limbic, 2023). It analyzes patient responses during initial assessments and suggests appropriate care pathways. That's AI making clinical decisions—or at least recommendations—before you ever meet the patient.

Crisis helplines increasingly use **natural language processing** algorithms to detect suicide risk in real-time conversations. Some trusts have implemented **predictive analytics** systems that flag patients at high risk of relapse based on patterns in electronic health records (Graham et al., 2019). Community mental health teams use scheduling algorithms that consider dozens of variables—patient acuity, geographical location, appointment history—to optimize caseload management.

You might not see the code running in the background. You just see the risk score on your screen, the appointment suggestion in your calendar, or the recommended intervention in the care plan template. But make no mistake: AI is shaping clinical decisions in ways that would have seemed impossible a decade ago.

The problem? Most mental health nurses received zero training on how these systems work, what their limitations are, or when to trust them versus when to override them. You're expected to integrate AI recommendations into your clinical judgment without understanding the evidence base, the potential for bias, or the legal implications when things go wrong.

That stops here.

The Nurse's Dilemma: Drowning in Admin While Patients Wait

Let's talk about your actual workday. You arrive at 9 a.m. with 12 patients on your caseload who need face-to-face contact this week. By 9:30 a.m., you've already spent 20 minutes documenting yesterday's visits, responding to three urgent emails, and updating risk assessments in the electronic system that crashes twice before saving your work.

A patient calls in crisis at 10 a.m. You spend 45 minutes on the phone doing a thorough risk assessment, de-escalating their distress, and arranging an earlier appointment. Then you spend another 20 minutes documenting the call, updating the care plan, notifying the duty consultant, and sending referral information to the crisis team—just in case.

By lunchtime, you've seen one patient face-to-face. You have seven more scheduled this week, plus two home visits that will take up most of Friday. You still need to complete monthly reviews for four patients, attend an MDT meeting tomorrow, and somehow find time to actually read the NICE guidance on that new treatment protocol your manager mentioned last month.

This is the reality: **administrative burden** consumes 40-60% of clinical time in community mental health settings (Royal College of Nursing, 2022). You're spending more time documenting care than delivering it. More time updating systems than building therapeutic relationships. More time in front of screens than in front of patients.

And you're exhausted. Not just tired—genuinely burned out. The kind of exhaustion that makes you question whether you can keep doing this job you once loved.

Now imagine if AI could handle the documentation. Not superficially, but actually write comprehensive, accurate notes while you focus on the patient. Imagine if predictive algorithms could identify which patients need urgent attention this week, allowing you to prioritize more effectively. Imagine if digital therapeutics could provide evidence-based interventions between your appointments, extending your reach without extending your hours.

That's not fantasy. That's what's already happening in some trusts. The gap between those who know how to leverage AI tools and those who don't is widening. This book exists to close that gap.

What This Book Will (and Won't) Do

This book will:

Demystify AI in plain language. No computer science degree required. You'll understand what machine learning actually means, how algorithms make predictions, and what "digital phenotyping" does beyond the buzzword. You'll learn enough technical context to have informed conversations with IT departments, vendors, and managers without feeling like you're faking fluency in a foreign language.

Show you exactly how to integrate AI tools into your workflow. Not theory. Not "someday we might." You'll get practical guidance on using AI for documentation, interpreting risk calculators, prescribing digital therapeutics, and managing the blended care model where technology supplements (not replaces) human contact.

Prepare you for the ethical challenges. AI brings thorny questions about privacy, bias, accountability, and the therapeutic relationship. We'll explore real scenarios where algorithms failed, examine the potential for AI to amplify health inequalities, and discuss your professional responsibility when you disagree with what the machine recommends.

Give you the evidence. Every claim in this book is backed by research. You'll learn what NICE and NHS England actually say about digital interventions, which apps have solid evidence bases, and where the gaps in research leave us making educated guesses rather than evidence-based decisions.

Position you as an advocate. You're not just a user of AI systems—you're the clinical expert who knows when they help and when they harm. This book will help you articulate concerns, push back on poorly implemented technology, and advocate for tools that genuinely serve patients rather than just generate impressive data for trust boards.

This book won't:

Teach you to code. You don't need to write algorithms to use them effectively, any more than you need to understand combustion engines to drive a car. We'll focus on what you need to know to be clinically competent, not technically expert.

Replace your clinical judgment. AI augments human expertise; it doesn't substitute for it. This book assumes you're already a competent mental health nurse. We're adding tools to your skillset, not replacing the skills you already have.

Claim AI solves everything. Technology is not a magic solution to systemic problems like underfunding, understaffing, or inadequate community resources. We'll be honest about what AI can and cannot do, and critical about implementations that prioritize efficiency over quality of care.

Pretend there are easy answers. AI in healthcare raises profound questions about autonomy, privacy, equity, and what it means to provide compassionate care in an increasingly digital world. We'll explore these dilemmas thoughtfully, not offer simplistic reassurances.

How to Use This Book: Choose Your Own Journey

This book is designed for flexibility. You can read cover to cover, but you don't have to. Here's how to navigate based on your needs:

If you're new to AI entirely: Start with Part 1 (Chapters 1.0-3.0). These chapters build your foundational understanding without assuming prior knowledge. You'll learn the terminology, understand the main types of AI in mental health, and get oriented to the landscape before moving into practical applications.

If you're drowning in admin: Jump straight to Chapter 4.0. This chapter focuses specifically on using AI to reclaim your time—documentation tools, scheduling systems, and workflow optimization. You can always circle back to the conceptual foundations later.

If you're already using AI tools but feeling uncertain: Go to Chapter 5.0 on AI-enhanced diagnostics, then Chapter 8.0 on data governance and ethics. You need to understand how to interpret AI outputs and when to trust them, plus the legal and ethical framework around your use of these systems.

If you want to prescribe digital therapeutics: Chapter 6.0 is your starting point. It covers everything from the evidence base to the practical conversation with patients about using apps as part of their care plan. Follow up with Chapter 3.0 to understand the DTx landscape more broadly.

If you're worried about getting it wrong: Chapter 11.0 addresses accountability, liability, and what happens when AI makes mistakes. This is essential reading if you're concerned about professional indemnity or NMC standards.

If you're a manager or clinical lead: Read Chapters 7.0, 9.0, 10.0, and 13.0. These cover implementation case studies, addressing algorithmic bias, building patient trust, and creating effective implementation strategies. Chapter 13.0 gives you the 90-day roadmap for rolling out AI in your service.

By role:

Community Psychiatric Nurses: Chapters 4.0, 5.0, 6.0, and 8.0 are essential. Focus on workflow integration, risk assessment, prescribing DTx, and privacy concerns.

Nurse Managers: Chapters 7.0, 9.0, 11.0, 13.0, and 14.0. You need implementation strategies, equity considerations, legal frameworks, and resources for team training.

Nurse Informaticists: Start with Chapters 1.0, 2.0, 8.0, and 9.0 to understand the technical foundations and data governance issues. Then read Chapters 13.0 and 14.0 for implementation and staying current.

Crisis/Acute Care Nurses: Chapters 2.0, 5.0, and 10.0. Digital phenotyping, AI diagnostics, and building trust in crisis situations are particularly relevant to your context.

Throughout the book, you'll find:

Case examples drawn from real clinical situations (with identifying details changed). These illustrate both successes and failures, because you learn as much from what went wrong as what went right.

Practical tools including decision trees, conversation scripts, evaluation templates, and checklists you can actually use in practice.

Red flags highlighting when to be skeptical, when to seek additional input, and when to override the algorithm entirely.

Evidence summaries giving you the research backing (or lack thereof) for different approaches, tools, and claims.

Reflection questions to help you think through how concepts apply to your specific context, patients, and practice setting.

The goal is simple: by the time you finish this book, you'll be confident using AI tools, competent in evaluating new technologies, and equipped to advocate for implementations that genuinely improve patient care while protecting the therapeutic relationship that remains at the heart of mental health nursing.

AI is here. It's time to understand it, use it effectively, and shape how it develops in ways that serve patients and practitioners rather than just administrators and algorithms.

Chapter 1.0: AI Demystified

You've probably heard a dozen different definitions of **artificial intelligence**, most of them either terrifyingly dystopian or irritatingly vague. Let's cut through the confusion. AI isn't magic, it isn't sentient, and it isn't coming for your job (though it might change how you do it). At its core, AI is pattern recognition at scale—systems that learn from data to make predictions or decisions without being explicitly programmed for every scenario.

Think of it this way: traditional computer programs follow rigid if-then rules. If temperature exceeds 38°C, then flag as fever. If patient reports suicidal ideation, then assess risk. Every possibility has to be anticipated and coded in advance.

AI works differently. You feed the system thousands of examples—patient records, symptom patterns, treatment outcomes—and it identifies relationships you might not have noticed. It learns that certain combinations of sleep disruption, social withdrawal, and specific word choices in clinical notes often precede relapse. It doesn't know *why* these patterns exist. It just recognizes them with increasing accuracy as it processes more data.

That's both the power and the peril of AI. It can spot patterns invisible to human observers, but it can also perpetuate biases hidden in training data or make predictions based on correlations that don't reflect causation. Understanding the distinction between what AI can and cannot do is essential for using it safely and effectively.

1.1 What AI Actually Is

Strip away the Hollywood dramatics and the breathless tech journalism, and AI is fundamentally about automation and optimization. These systems automate tasks that previously required human intelligence—recognizing speech, interpreting images, predicting outcomes, generating text. They optimize by finding patterns in data far too large for human analysis.

Artificial intelligence refers to any computer system that can perform tasks typically requiring human intelligence (Russell & Norvig, 2020). That's a deliberately broad definition, encompassing everything from the spam filter in your email to the sophisticated algorithms recommending patient interventions.

In healthcare, AI manifests in three main ways: systems that **predict** future events (like which patients are at risk of crisis), systems that **generate** content (like drafting clinical documentation), and systems that **interact** with patients directly (like therapeutic chatbots). Each type serves different clinical functions and carries different risks.

What AI is *not*: It's not conscious. It's not creative in the human sense. It doesn't "understand" mental illness the way you understand it after sitting with a patient through their darkest moments. AI processes patterns in data. It doesn't grasp meaning, feel empathy, or exercise the kind of holistic clinical judgment that comes from years of experience (Topol, 2019).

Here's where this matters clinically: An AI risk calculator might flag a patient as high risk based on documented risk factors, but it won't know that the patient mentioned they're going on holiday next week—a protective factor not captured in structured data fields. It won't pick up on the subtle shift in tone that tells you someone is actually doing better despite similar symptom scores. It won't recognize when a patient is telling you what they think you want to hear.

That's why the future of mental health care isn't AI *or* nurses. It's AI *and* nurses—what researchers call the **"centaur model"** of human-machine collaboration, where each contributes what they do best (Topol, 2019). AI handles pattern recognition in vast datasets. You bring contextual understanding, therapeutic relationship, and the kind of judgment that can't be reduced to an algorithm.

1.2 Predictive AI Tools

Predictive AI uses historical data to forecast future events. In mental health nursing, this typically means risk calculators, early warning systems, and tools that identify patients who need escalated care before crisis occurs.

The technology works by analyzing patterns in electronic health records, demographic information, treatment history, and sometimes behavioral data. The algorithm learns which combinations of factors historically preceded adverse events—suicide attempts, hospital admissions, disengagement from services, violent incidents—and flags current patients showing similar patterns (Graham et al., 2019).

NHS trusts increasingly deploy these tools for suicide risk prediction, though the evidence base remains mixed. A 2019 study analyzing data from over 5,000 patients found that machine learning algorithms predicted suicide attempts with modest accuracy—better than chance, but far from perfect (Belsher et al., 2019). The algorithm correctly identified about 30% of patients who went on to attempt suicide, while flagging many others who didn't.

Think about what that means clinically. You're reviewing your caseload, and the system flags Maria (not her real name) as high risk. The algorithm noted that she recently restarted antidepressants after a gap in treatment, missed two appointments last month, and has multiple previous admissions. All accurate. All concerning.

But the algorithm doesn't know that Maria missed appointments because she started a new job with inflexible hours—a positive development. It doesn't know she restarted medication proactively after recognizing early warning signs, demonstrating improved self-awareness. It doesn't know her sister just moved nearby, expanding her support network.

You need the algorithm's pattern recognition. It caught something you might have missed while managing 12 other patients. But you also need your clinical judgment to interpret what the pattern actually means in this specific person's life right now.

Early warning systems take prediction a step further, monitoring multiple data streams for concerning changes. Some systems track medication adherence through electronic prescribing data. Others analyze the tone and content of patient messages in secure messaging platforms. More sophisticated implementations integrate data from multiple sources—appointment attendance, crisis line contacts, hospital admissions, even social media activity if patients consent (Torous et al., 2018).

The King's College London group developed a system that identifies patients at risk of disengaging from early intervention in psychosis services by analyzing patterns in appointment attendance, medication collection, and clinical notes (Koutsouleris et al., 2016). The algorithm predicts disengagement up to six months in advance with reasonable accuracy, potentially allowing intervention before patients drop out of care entirely.

Here's the crucial part: these tools work best when integrated into clinical workflow, not as separate systems requiring additional data entry. If you have to input information twice—once in your documentation system and again in a risk calculator—you probably won't use it consistently. Effective implementations pull data from existing electronic records and present predictions at natural decision points, like when you're preparing for an appointment or reviewing weekly caseload prioritization.

1.3 Generative AI Applications

Generative AI creates new content—text, images, even synthetic voices. In mental health nursing, the primary application is documentation assistance, though the technology is expanding rapidly.

You know the drill. You spend 30 minutes with a patient conducting a thorough mental state examination. Then you spend another 20 minutes documenting the encounter, trying to capture everything clinically relevant while meeting documentation standards, satisfying audit requirements, and writing clearly enough that the duty psychiatrist can understand the situation at 2 a.m. tomorrow when they're reviewing your patient's crisis presentation.

Generative AI tools promise to change this. **Ambient clinical intelligence** systems use natural language processing to listen to your conversation with the patient (with their consent), identify clinically relevant information, and automatically generate draft documentation (Quiroz et al., 2019).

The technology isn't perfect. Early versions required significant editing and couldn't reliably distinguish between information the patient shared and questions you asked. Current systems are improving. They can generate reasonably accurate progress notes, though you still need to review and refine them (Cheng et al., 2021).

Some NHS trusts are piloting systems where you dictate notes immediately after appointments using voice recognition software enhanced with AI. The algorithm knows medical terminology, understands clinical context, and can structure your spoken words into proper documentation format. What used to take 20 minutes now takes five—mostly spent reviewing for accuracy rather than typing.

But here's what worries clinicians (and should worry you): if AI writes your notes, are you actually thinking through the clinical picture as thoroughly? Documentation isn't just bureaucratic box-ticking. It's part of clinical reasoning. The act of organizing your observations into coherent notes helps you notice patterns, identify gaps, and formulate plans (Poissant et al., 2005).

There's a balance to strike. AI can handle the tedious parts—formatting, structure, pulling in relevant history from previous notes. You still need to do the thinking. The technology should reduce administrative burden without reducing clinical reflection.

Other generative AI applications include drafting patient communications, creating educational materials tailored to individual patients' literacy levels, and generating care plan templates based on evidence-based protocols. The NHS is exploring AI-generated reminders for appointments, medication adherence prompts, and even automated responses to common patient queries in secure messaging systems (NHS England, 2023).

The ethical question hovering over all of this: when does efficient automation cross into something that feels less personal, less human? If your appointment reminder comes from an algorithm, does that matter? What about if the response to your crisis message comes from AI? Where's the line?

1.4 Therapeutic AI Systems

Here's where it gets really interesting—and controversial. **Therapeutic AI** systems don't just support your clinical work; they interact directly with patients, providing interventions without human involvement (or with minimal human oversight).

The most common form is **chatbot therapy**. These are conversational agents that conduct structured therapeutic interactions via text or voice interface. They're not replacing therapy in the traditional sense. They're providing scalable access to evidence-based techniques for people who wouldn't otherwise receive any intervention.

Wysa, one of the most widely deployed mental health chatbots, has been used by over 5 million people globally, including through NHS pilots (Inkster et al., 2018). The system offers cognitive-behavioral techniques, mindfulness exercises, and crisis support through a conversational interface. Research shows modest but significant improvements in anxiety and depression symptoms for users who engage consistently (Inkster et al., 2018).

Think about what this means for your patients on waiting lists. Someone contacts your service seeking help for anxiety. The wait for first assessment is eight weeks. Traditionally, they get nothing in the interim except maybe a leaflet and a crisis number. Now they might get access to a chatbot that teaches breathing exercises, helps them identify cognitive distortions, and provides basic support while they wait.

That's not replacing your work. It's providing something rather than nothing during a gap in care.

Digital therapeutics more broadly include apps and platforms delivering structured interventions. **Sleepio** provides digital CBT for insomnia and has demonstrated effectiveness comparable to face-to-face therapy in randomized controlled trials (Espie et al., 2019). **Deprexis** offers 10 modules of CBT for depression, with research showing significant symptom reduction (Berger et al., 2011).

These aren't wellness apps with affirmations and mood tracking. They're regulated medical devices delivering evidence-based protocols. The distinction matters for clinical accountability, which we'll explore thoroughly in Chapter 3.0.

Some therapeutic AI systems operate more autonomously. **Woebot**, another chatbot therapist, uses AI to adapt its responses based on how users interact over time. It tracks mood patterns, identifies concerning changes, and adjusts the therapeutic approach accordingly (Fitzpatrick et al., 2017). When the system detects crisis indicators, it escalates to human support.

The technology raises profound questions. Can an algorithm form a therapeutic alliance? Does it matter if patients improve despite having no relationship with a human therapist? What gets lost when we automate aspects of care that have always been fundamentally relational?

I don't have definitive answers to these questions. Neither does anyone else, honestly. We're in the middle of a massive, uncontrolled experiment in what happens when technology mediates mental health care. Your role as a clinician is to think critically about these implementations, evaluate outcomes rigorously, and advocate for approaches that genuinely serve patients rather than just reducing costs.

1.5 Understanding the Technology

You don't need to know how to build these systems, but you do need to understand what's happening under the hood well enough to evaluate their limitations. Three terms come up constantly: **machine learning**, **deep learning**, and **natural language processing**. Here's what they actually mean.

Machine learning (ML) is the umbrella term for systems that improve their performance through experience rather than explicit programming. You give the algorithm a dataset with inputs and desired outputs (e.g., patient symptoms and diagnoses), and it learns to map inputs to outputs by identifying patterns (Mitchell, 1997). Once trained, it can make predictions on new data it hasn't seen before.

There are different types. **Supervised learning** uses labeled data—you tell the system which patients developed depression, and it learns to identify features predicting depression in others. **Unsupervised learning** finds patterns without being told what to look for—it might cluster patients into groups based on symptom profiles without predetermined categories. **Reinforcement learning** learns through trial and error, like how a chatbot improves by tracking which responses lead to positive user engagement (Russell & Norvig, 2020).

Deep learning is a specialized form of machine learning using neural networks with multiple layers, loosely inspired by how the brain processes information. These systems excel at tasks like image recognition (analyzing brain scans) and language understanding (interpreting clinical notes). They can handle much more complex patterns than traditional machine learning but require enormous amounts of training data and computing power (LeCun et al., 2015).

The "deep" refers to layers of processing. An algorithm analyzing your documentation might have one layer that identifies individual words, another that recognizes phrases, another that understands sentence structure, and another that grasps overall meaning and clinical significance. Each layer builds on the previous one.

Natural language processing (NLP) enables computers to understand human language. This powers everything from voice-to-text documentation to chatbots that interpret patient messages. NLP algorithms can extract structured information from unstructured text, like identifying mentions of suicidal ideation in clinical notes or detecting sentiment changes in patient communications (Hirschberg & Manning, 2015).

Here's why this matters: When you use an AI tool, understanding which type of technology powers it helps you anticipate its limitations. Machine learning systems need large, high-quality training datasets—if trained primarily on one population, they may perform poorly on others. Deep learning excels at complex patterns but operates as a "black box" where even developers can't fully explain why it made specific predictions. NLP systems can be thrown off by ambiguous language, sarcasm, or cultural idioms.

You're not expected to audit the algorithms. But knowing that an AI risk calculator uses supervised learning tells you to ask: what data was it trained on? How diverse was that population? How recent is the data? These aren't technical questions—they're clinical questions about whether the tool is appropriate for your patients.

1.6 Why Nurses Matter Most

Data scientists can build algorithms. Programmers can write code. Technology companies can deploy systems at scale. But none of them can tell whether these tools actually work in real clinical practice. That's where you come in.

You're the bridge between technology and patients. You know what actually happens when someone is in crisis at 3 a.m. You understand the subtle communication that builds trust with someone who's spent years avoiding mental health services. You recognize when documentation requirements conflict with therapeutic presence. You see how socioeconomic factors, cultural background, and lived experience shape how people engage with services.

AI developers typically don't have this knowledge. They optimize for metrics that don't capture what matters clinically. An algorithm might be 80% accurate at predicting hospital admission, but if it achieves that accuracy by flagging every patient with previous admissions—regardless of current clinical picture—it's not actually useful. You're the one who knows that (Graham et al., 2019).

Implementation success depends on frontline nurses more than technical sophistication. Research consistently shows that the biggest barriers to effective health IT adoption aren't technological—they're workflow integration, user acceptance, and alignment with clinical priorities (Bates et al., 2014). You can have the most accurate AI system in the world, but if it adds three clicks to your documentation process or presents information in ways that don't match how you actually make decisions, you won't use it consistently.

Here's what effective implementation looks like: developers work *with* clinicians from the beginning, not just at the end. Nurses help define the problems worth solving, identify points in workflow where AI could genuinely help, test prototypes in real clinical contexts, and provide honest feedback about what works and what doesn't. The technology adapts to clinical practice, not the other way around (Shaw et al., 2019).

You're also the ones who catch problems before they harm patients. An algorithm flagging low-risk patients as high-risk wastes resources but probably won't cause direct harm. An algorithm missing high-risk patients absolutely can. You're the safety net. You notice when predictions don't match clinical reality. You override the algorithm when your assessment suggests something different.

You escalate concerns about bias, accuracy, or inappropriate implementation.

The risk is that AI becomes a tool for deskilling—making clinical decisions more standardized, more protocol-driven, less dependent on expertise (Topol, 2019). The opportunity is that AI becomes a tool for upskilling—freeing you from administrative burden so you can focus on the complex, nuanced work that genuinely requires human judgment.

Which path we take depends largely on whether nurses are involved in shaping how AI is deployed. If implementation is driven by IT departments focused on efficiency metrics and trust leadership focused on cost savings, we'll likely get the former. If implementation is led by clinicians who understand both the potential and the pitfalls, we have a chance at the latter.

1.7 Moving Forward Equipped

Understanding AI isn't optional anymore. These systems are shaping clinical decisions, influencing resource allocation, and changing how patients experience care. You need enough literacy to evaluate whether tools are evidence-based, recognize when they're working poorly, and advocate for implementations that genuinely improve practice.

The following chapters build on these foundations. You'll learn how specific technologies work, how to integrate them into workflow, and how to navigate the ethical challenges that inevitably arise. You'll see case examples of both successful implementations and instructive failures. You'll get practical tools for evaluating new systems and frameworks for having difficult conversations about privacy, bias, and accountability.

AI in mental health nursing is still evolving rapidly. The tools available next year will be more sophisticated than what exists today. But the fundamental principles don't change: technology should serve clinical goals, not dictate them. Algorithms should augment human judgment, not substitute for it. Efficiency matters, but not more than quality of care and the therapeutic relationship.

You're not becoming a data scientist. You're becoming a clinician who can use data science tools effectively, critically, and ethically. That's an essential skillset for practicing mental health nursing in the 21st century.

Chapter 2.0: Digital Phenotyping Explained

Your patient's smartphone knows things about their mental state that they might not tell you. It knows when they stopped getting out of bed until noon. It knows their social interactions dropped by 80% over three weeks. It knows they're searching "how to cope with depression" at 2 a.m. more frequently.

This is **digital phenotyping**—using data from personal digital devices to characterize behavior patterns relevant to mental health (Torous et al., 2016). The technology passively collects information from smartphones, wearables, and other devices to create a detailed picture of someone's daily functioning without requiring them to fill out questionnaires or remember to track symptoms.

It sounds intrusive because it absolutely can be. It also sounds potentially valuable because it absolutely is. The challenge is figuring out when the benefits justify the privacy concerns, how to implement it ethically, and what to do with the data once you have it.

2.1 Your Phone as Monitor

Let's start with what's actually being collected. **Digital phenotyping** relies on passive data streams—information generated automatically through device use rather than actively reported by the patient (Onnela & Rauch, 2016).

Accelerometer data tracks movement patterns. How much is someone moving throughout the day? When do they get up? When do they go to bed? How does their activity level compare to their baseline? Research shows that reduced physical activity often precedes depressive episodes, while increased agitation might signal emerging mania (Saeb et al., 2015).

GPS location data reveals mobility and routine. Are they leaving the house? Visiting their usual places? Breaking established patterns? Social isolation manifests as smaller "life space"—the geographical area someone regularly inhabits. Studies demonstrate that people experiencing depression show significantly reduced mobility compared to their baseline (Saeb et al., 2015).

Communication metadata tracks phone calls and messages without accessing content. How often is someone communicating? Who are they contacting? Has their social network suddenly contracted? You don't need to read messages to detect concerning patterns. The frequency, timing, and variability of communication provide meaningful signals (Saeb et al., 2017).

Screen time and app usage show engagement patterns. Excessive smartphone use might indicate avoidance behaviors. Obsessive checking of certain apps could signal anxiety. Dramatic increases in screen time during usual sleep hours might indicate insomnia or nighttime rumination (Abdullah et al., 2016).

Keyboard dynamics analyze typing patterns. Speed, accuracy, pause length, and autocorrect usage change during mood episodes. Research at the University of Copenhagen found that typing behavior predicts depressive symptoms with reasonable accuracy (Zulueta et al., 2018). People type more slowly and make more errors when depressed. They type faster and more impulsively during manic episodes.

Voice analysis detects changes in speech patterns. Pitch, tempo, energy levels, and word choice shift with mental state. Some systems can identify depression from 30-second voice samples with accuracy comparable to clinical interviews (Cummins et al., 2015). This isn't about *what* you say—it's about *how* you say it.

The technology aggregates these data streams into **digital biomarkers**—quantifiable behavioral indicators of mental state. Think of them like vital signs for mental health, except instead of measuring heart rate and blood pressure, you're measuring social engagement, circadian patterns, and activity levels.

2.2 Digital Biomarkers Demystified

Not all data is equally useful. Effective digital phenotyping focuses on behaviors with validated connections to clinical outcomes. Four categories show the strongest evidence: **activity patterns**, **sleep/circadian rhythms**, **social behavior**, and **mobility**.

Activity patterns reflect energy levels and motivation. The relationship between physical activity and mood is well-established (Schuch et al., 2018). Digital phenotyping can track this continuously and objectively, unlike self-reported questionnaires that rely on memory and subjective perception.

A study at Northwestern University followed people with bipolar disorder for three months using smartphone sensors (Beiwinkel et al., 2016). The algorithm detected manic episodes an average of 6 days before clinical diagnosis by identifying increased movement, irregular sleep-wake patterns, and higher communication frequency. It caught depressive episodes about 7 days early through decreased movement and social withdrawal.

That's potentially game-changing. Early intervention during prodromal symptoms generally produces better outcomes than treatment after full relapse (Birchwood et al., 2013). If technology can flag concerning changes before clinical threshold, you might prevent crisis rather than just responding to it.

Sleep and circadian patterns are both symptoms and predictors of mental health problems. Insomnia increases risk of depression onset. Disrupted sleep precedes mood episodes in bipolar disorder. Irregular sleep-wake patterns correlate with anxiety (Harvey, 2008).

Digital phenotyping captures this through accelerometer data showing when someone is stationary for extended periods, combined with screen use patterns. You can identify not just sleep duration but consistency, which often matters more clinically than total hours (Bouwmans et al., 2018).

Social behavior provides insight into engagement and connection. Humans are fundamentally social. Isolation predicts poor outcomes across virtually every mental health condition. Digital phenotyping quantifies this through communication frequency, response time to messages, and diversity of contacts (Saeb et al., 2017).

Elena, a 34-year-old woman with recurrent depression (composite case), had been stable for 18 months. Her digital phenotyping data showed gradual but consistent changes over four weeks: 45% reduction in communication frequency, 60% decrease in distinct contacts, increased nighttime phone use, and reduced daytime movement. Her mood self-reports during this period remained relatively stable—she wasn't aware her behavior was changing significantly.

Her CPN received an automated alert about declining social engagement. During their next check-in, focused assessment revealed early depressive symptoms Elena had been minimizing. They increased therapy frequency and adjusted her care plan proactively. Elena didn't reach crisis. She didn't require admission. The technology spotted a pattern she couldn't see herself.

Mobility patterns show how much physical space someone occupies in their daily life. Reduced mobility—spending most time at home, visiting fewer locations, traveling shorter distances—correlates strongly with depression severity (Canzian & Musolesi, 2015). The relationship is bidirectional: depression reduces motivation to leave home, and staying home worsens mood through decreased social contact, reduced sunlight exposure, and disrupted routine.

GPS data can track this automatically. You're not watching where patients go—that would be unacceptably intrusive. You're measuring how much their "life space" has expanded or contracted compared to their personal baseline.

2.3 When Technology Predicts Crisis

Here's where digital phenotyping moves from interesting to potentially lifesaving. Can we predict suicide attempts, psychotic episodes, or other crises before they occur?

The evidence is emerging but not yet definitive. A 2020 study at Mindstrong Health tracked 126 people with serious mental illness using smartphone sensors for six months (Huckvale et al., 2019). The algorithm predicted psychiatric hospitalization 6-14 days in advance with 70-80% accuracy by detecting changes in activity, sleep, mobility, and phone use patterns.

That's far from perfect. Twenty to thirty percent of hospitalizations weren't predicted. The system also generated false alarms—people flagged as high risk who didn't deteriorate. But here's the important question: is 70% prediction better than the alternative? Without any predictive system, you're essentially waiting for patients to present in crisis or hoping they'll recognize warning signs and contact services proactively.

Suicide prediction is particularly challenging and ethically fraught. Machine learning algorithms analyzing social media posts can identify suicide risk with modest accuracy (Coppersmith et al., 2018). Systems monitoring search history and typing patterns show similar results. But the base rate problem makes this difficult: suicide attempts are relatively rare events, so even accurate algorithms generate many false positives for every true positive identified.

Imagine your service implements suicide prediction software. It analyzes patient data continuously and flags 10 people this month as high risk. Three are genuinely at elevated risk. Seven are false alarms. You can't know which is which, so you contact all 10 for urgent assessment.

Is that beneficial? You've potentially caught three people heading toward crisis. You've also disrupted care for seven others, possibly causing distress by suddenly treating them as high risk when they weren't. And what about the patients *not* flagged who still attempt? Did the technology lull you into false confidence about them?

These aren't rhetorical questions. They're real dilemmas facing mental health services implementing predictive technologies right now. Research suggests careful implementation can be beneficial, but only when combined with appropriate clinical response protocols and clear communication with patients about how the technology works (Torous & Roberts, 2017).

Psychosis detection shows more promise with fewer ethical landmines. Speech patterns change in prodromal psychosis—responses become more tangential, thought processes more disorganized, word choices more abstract (Corcoran et al., 2018). Analysis of voice recordings can identify these changes before florid symptoms emerge.

The University of California developed a system analyzing brief voice samples from young people at clinical high risk for psychosis (Corcoran et al., 2018). The algorithm predicted conversion to psychosis up to two years in advance with 80% accuracy. That's remarkable. Early intervention in psychosis dramatically improves long-term outcomes (Fusar-Poli et al., 2017). If technology can identify who will develop psychosis before it's clinically obvious, we can target intensive intervention to those who need it most.

2.4 The Consent Conversation

You can't just start monitoring patient data without explicit, informed consent. This isn't optional. It's legal requirement, ethical imperative, and clinical common sense. The conversation needs to cover what's being collected, how it's used, who has access, how long it's stored, and crucially—what happens when the system detects problems.

Here's how that conversation might go with a patient named Marcus (composite case) who has bipolar disorder:

You: "We're piloting a program that uses smartphone data to help identify early warning signs of mood episodes. I want to explain how it works and see if you'd be interested."

Marcus: "What do you mean by smartphone data?"

You: "The app runs in the background on your phone and tracks things like how much you're moving around, your sleep patterns, and general communication frequency—how often you're texting or calling people. It doesn't access any content—I can't see your messages or know who you're talking to. It's measuring patterns of behavior."

Marcus: "So you're watching me?"

You: "Not exactly. The system looks for changes in your patterns compared to your own baseline. If your activity suddenly increases a lot, or your sleep becomes irregular, or your social contact drops significantly, it creates an alert for me to check in with you. The goal is to catch mood episodes early, maybe even before you notice yourself."

Marcus: "What if I don't want you to see all that?"

You: "Then you don't participate. This is completely voluntary. Your care doesn't change if you say no."

Marcus: "Who else can see this information?"

You: "Only your direct care team—me and the psychiatrist who prescribes your medication. It's stored securely within NHS systems. The technology company that makes the app can see anonymized data for research and improvement, but they won't know who you are."

Marcus: "What happens if the system thinks I'm getting manic? Do I have to come in immediately?"

You: "Good question. If we get an alert, I'll contact you—usually by phone—to check in and see how you're doing. We'd decide together whether you need to come in or if we can manage it remotely. The system doesn't force anything. It's just early warning information that supplements our regular check-ins."

This conversation needs to be documented thoroughly. UK consent standards require patients understand what they're agreeing to, including potential risks (GMC, 2020). The main risk here isn't that monitoring harms them directly—it's that it might create anxiety about being watched, alter their behavior because they know they're being tracked, or generate false alarms leading to unnecessary interventions.

Some patients find digital monitoring reassuring. They like having an additional safety net. Others find it infantilizing or intrusive. Both responses are valid. Your job is to explain accurately without pressure.

Special populations require extra consideration. Young people under 18 need parental consent in most circumstances, though mature minors can sometimes consent independently. People with impaired capacity need decisions made in their best interest, ideally with involvement from lasting power of attorney or family. Patients in forensic settings may have different consent requirements depending on whether monitoring is court-mandated or voluntary (Mental Capacity Act, 2005).

2.5 Ethical Boundaries Explained

Digital phenotyping sits at the uncomfortable intersection of beneficial monitoring and unwelcome surveillance. Here's where the lines get drawn.

Red flag #1: Monitoring without ongoing consent. Consent isn't one-time. It's continuous. Just because someone agreed to monitoring six months ago doesn't mean they still agree now. Best practice includes regular check-ins about whether patients want to continue, easy ways to opt out at any time, and mechanisms for patients to request deletion of collected data (Huckvale et al., 2019).

Red flag #2: Using data for purposes beyond direct clinical care. If you collect data to monitor mental health, you can't suddenly start using it for other purposes—even well-intentioned ones. Analyzing patient location data to study healthcare access patterns, for example, would require separate consent even if anonymized (Vayena et al., 2015).

Red flag #3: Sharing data beyond the immediate care team. Insurance companies would love access to digital phenotyping data for risk assessment. Researchers want it for studies. Employers might claim they need it for occupational health reasons. The answer to all of these is no unless patients provide explicit consent for each specific use (Huckvale et al., 2019).

Red flag #4: Algorithmic decision-making without human oversight. An automated system that contacts emergency services when it detects crisis indicators sounds efficient. It's also terrifying. What if it's wrong? What if the "crisis" is actually someone staying up late watching movies? Algorithms inform human decisions; they shouldn't make them autonomously (Torous & Roberts, 2017).

Red flag #5: Asymmetric access to data. If you're collecting patient data, patients should be able to see it. Transparency builds trust. Patients have the right to know what's being recorded about them and how it's being interpreted. Systems that give clinicians data access while keeping patients in the dark are ethically problematic (Martinez-Martin et al., 2018).

Red flag #6: Ignoring digital inequity. Not everyone has a smartphone. Not everyone has unlimited data. Not everyone has technological literacy to use monitoring apps. If you implement digital phenotyping, you can't make it a prerequisite for accessing care. That would disadvantage already-marginalized populations (Torous et al., 2020).

A Bradford trust piloted digital phenotyping for early intervention in psychosis (composite example). Young people were given smartphones with pre-loaded monitoring apps. Participation was voluntary. After six months, clinicians reviewed the program. They found concerning disparities: young people from affluent areas engaged consistently, while those from deprived areas had erratic participation despite similar mental health needs.

Why? Some couldn't afford data plans even with free phones. Others had chaotic home situations where phones got lost or stolen. Some had immigration concerns making them wary of any surveillance technology. The program was technically successful but practically inequitable.

The trust adapted by offering Wi-Fi-only versions, allowing paper-based monitoring for those who declined digital options, and ensuring that opting out didn't affect care quality. Technology should expand access, not create new barriers.

2.6 Key Takeaways

Digital phenotyping offers something genuinely new in mental health care: continuous, objective measurement of behavior patterns that correlate with clinical outcomes. Instead of relying entirely on patient self-report during weekly or monthly check-ins, you can detect changes as they happen.

The technology isn't perfect. Algorithms miss some relapses and flag false alarms regularly. Privacy concerns are substantial and legitimate. Implementation requires careful attention to consent, equity, and appropriate use of data.

But for some patients, in some contexts, digital phenotyping might prevent crisis, enable earlier intervention, and provide reassurance that someone's paying attention even between appointments. That's worth exploring carefully and ethically.

Your role as a mental health nurse isn't to become a data analyst. It's to understand what digital phenotyping can and cannot tell you, to use insights appropriately within clinical judgment, and to advocate for implementations that respect patients while leveraging technology's potential.

The next chapter examines another category of digital tools—not monitoring but treatment itself through digital therapeutics.

-Chapter 3.0: Digital Therapeutics

You can now prescribe an app. Not in the casual sense of recommending someone download a meditation tracker—in the medical sense of prescribing a regulated therapeutic intervention with evidence demonstrating clinical efficacy.

Digital therapeutics (DTx) are evidence-based therapeutic interventions delivered via software to prevent, manage, or treat medical conditions (Digital Therapeutics Alliance, 2021). They're not wellness apps. They're not mood trackers with inspirational quotes. They're medical devices subject to regulatory approval, evaluated through clinical trials, and held to standards similar to pharmaceutical treatments.

This changes your practice. You're no longer limited to face-to-face contact and medication. You can prescribe structured interventions—cognitive-behavioral therapy, exposure therapy, sleep restriction protocols—delivered digitally between your appointments. You can extend your therapeutic reach without extending your hours. You can offer evidence-based treatment to people on waiting lists rather than leaving them with nothing.

But prescribing DTx isn't as simple as telling someone to download an app. You need to understand the evidence base, match interventions to patients appropriately, set realistic expectations, and monitor outcomes. This chapter gives you the framework to do that competently.

3.1 Evidence and Guidelines

Let's start with what the authorities actually say. **NICE guidance** on digital mental health interventions (NICE, 2022) recognizes computerized CBT and specific digital platforms as evidence-based options for mild-to-moderate depression and anxiety. They don't just acknowledge these tools exist—they actively recommend them as first-line treatment in appropriate cases.

NHS England's digital mental health strategy identifies DTx as essential for meeting demand with limited resources (NHS England, 2023). The Improving Access to Psychological Therapies (IAPT) program increasingly integrates digital options, recognizing that traditional face-to-face capacity can't meet population need.

The evidence base varies dramatically by condition and intervention. For **depression**, digital CBT platforms show consistent but modest effects. A 2017 meta-analysis of 20 randomized trials found guided internet-delivered CBT produced effect sizes of 0.67 compared to waitlist controls—statistically significant but smaller than face-to-face therapy (Karyotaki et al., 2017). Crucially, effectiveness depends heavily on whether there's human support. Fully automated programs show much smaller effects.

For **anxiety disorders**, the data is stronger. Digital CBT for generalized anxiety, social anxiety, and panic disorder demonstrates effects comparable to face-to-face treatment, particularly when combined with brief therapist contact (Andrews et al., 2018). Effect sizes range from 0.80 to 1.15 depending on the specific intervention and population.

Insomnia might be where digital therapeutics shine brightest. **Sleepio**, a digital CBT program for insomnia, has been studied in multiple large RCTs showing sustained improvements in sleep quality and duration (Espie et al., 2019). Effect sizes exceed many pharmacological treatments and persist at six-month follow-up. NICE explicitly recommends digital CBT-I as first-line treatment before considering medication.

The evidence for **serious mental illness** is much weaker. A few small studies show promise for digital interventions in psychosis or bipolar disorder, but sample sizes are tiny and follow-up is short

(Firth et al., 2017). These tools might have a role, but we don't yet know if they're helpful, harmful, or simply irrelevant for people with severe conditions.

What NICE doesn't recommend: replacing specialist care with apps, using DTx as sole treatment for moderate-to-severe conditions, or implementing platforms without adequate evidence. They emphasize that digital tools should be part of a care package, not substitutes for human contact when clinical need justifies it (NICE, 2022).

3.2 The Digital Treatment Landscape

The marketplace is crowded and confusing. Thousands of mental health apps exist. Most have zero evidence. Some make claims that range from overblown to fraudulent. Your job is separating legitimate therapeutics from expensive placebos.

Regulated digital therapeutics in the UK are designated as Class I or Class II medical devices under MHRA regulations (MHRA, 2023). This means they've undergone some level of regulatory review. It doesn't necessarily mean they're effective—regulatory approval focuses on safety and technical performance, not always clinical outcomes—but it's a baseline quality indicator.

The landscape breaks into several categories:

Self-contained CBT programs deliver structured cognitive-behavioral interventions without requiring therapist involvement. **Deprexis** is the archetype—10 modules covering behavioral activation, cognitive restructuring, mindfulness, social skills, and relapse prevention for depression (Berger et al., 2011). Users work through content at their own pace, complete exercises, and receive automated feedback. Research shows significant symptom reduction compared to waitlist, though effects are smaller than therapist-led treatment.

Guided digital interventions combine automated content with brief human support. **SilverCloud** provides CBT modules for depression, anxiety, and stress alongside weekly messages from a supporter who reviews progress and provides encouragement (Richards et al., 2020). The human element appears crucial—the same platform used without support shows much weaker effects. Patients need accountability, personalization, and the feeling that someone cares about their progress.

AI-powered chatbots provide conversational interactions that feel more personal than working through modules. **Wysa** engages users in text-based conversations, offering empathetic responses, teaching coping skills, and guiding CBT techniques through dialogue rather than didactic content (Inkster et al., 2018). The interface is appealing, particularly to young people comfortable with messaging. Evidence shows modest improvements in anxiety and depression, though effect sizes are smaller than guided interventions.

Condition-specific programs target particular problems. **Sleepio** for insomnia uses CBT-I techniques including sleep restriction, stimulus control, and cognitive therapy delivered through an animated therapist (Espie et al., 2019). **Daylight** focuses specifically on generalized anxiety using a blend of CBT and ACT principles (Huberty et al., 2021). **Pear Therapeutics** produces prescription digital therapeutics for substance use disorders approved in the United States though not yet widely available in the UK.

VR therapy platforms deliver exposure therapy through virtual environments. Someone with PTSD can gradually confront trauma-related stimuli in controlled virtual settings. Social anxiety can be treated through simulated social situations. Height phobia responds to virtual exposure at increasing heights. Evidence is promising but limited, and implementation requires VR hardware most patients don't own (Freeman et al., 2017).

Blended care platforms integrate digital and face-to-face treatment. You might see someone every other week, with digital content providing structure between sessions. You assign homework through the platform, review their progress remotely, and use appointments to address what emerged from their digital work. This model shows particularly strong outcomes (Erbe et al., 2017).

3.3 Popular Platforms Reviewed

Let's examine specific platforms you're likely to encounter. This isn't comprehensive—the landscape changes constantly—but these represent major players with established evidence.

Wysa: An empathetic chatbot providing CBT tools, mindfulness exercises, and emotional support. The interface feels conversational. The bot responds to mood check-ins with appropriate techniques—breathing exercises for anxiety, behavioral activation for low mood, thought challenging for rumination.

Strengths: Accessible 24/7. Engaging interface that feels less clinical than traditional CBT programs. Free tier with basic content. Evidence shows improvements in depression and anxiety scores for engaged users (Inkster et al., 2018).

Limitations: Fully automated with limited human support unless you pay for premium tiers. Can feel repetitive after extended use. Struggles with complex presentations. Best for mild symptoms or as adjunct to other treatment.

When to prescribe: Young adults with mild-to-moderate anxiety or depression who are comfortable with technology and messaging interfaces. Good option for people on waiting lists or as homework between sessions. Not appropriate for crisis situations despite marketing claims.

Sleepio: Digital CBT for insomnia delivered through an animated virtual therapist named "The Prof" who guides you through sleep restriction, stimulus control, and cognitive techniques over six weekly sessions.

Strengths: Strong evidence base with multiple large RCTs (Espie et al., 2019). Effects comparable to face-to-face CBT-I. NICE-recommended. Available on NHS prescription in some areas. Sustained improvements at long-term follow-up.

Limitations: Requires commitment to sleep restriction, which many people find difficult. Takes weeks to see improvement. Not suitable if insomnia is secondary to untreated mental illness or medical conditions. Expensive if self-paying.

When to prescribe: Primary insomnia without complex comorbidity. Patients motivated enough to track sleep diaries and follow protocols. Strong evidence supports using this before sleep medication. Works well as first-line treatment in mild-to-moderate cases.

Deprexis: Comprehensive digital CBT program for depression covering behavioral activation, cognitive restructuring, mindfulness, interpersonal skills, and relapse prevention across 10 modules.

Strengths: Thorough content based on established CBT protocols. Evidence from multiple RCTs showing symptom reduction (Berger et al., 2011). Can be used independently or alongside therapy. Covers range of techniques, so patients can focus on what's most relevant.

Limitations: Module-based format feels more like an online course than personalized therapy. Completion rates are modest—many people start but don't finish. Works better with therapist guidance than as standalone treatment.

When to prescribe: Moderate depression in people who prefer structured, self-directed approach. Works particularly well when you guide them through modules and review progress together. Good for people who've had CBT before and need refresher/extension.

Limbic Access: AI-powered triage and assessment tool primarily used by services rather than prescribed to patients. Analyzes responses during initial assessments to suggest appropriate care pathways.

Strengths: Reduces assessment burden. More consistent than human triage in some studies. Appears to reduce waiting times by routing patients efficiently (Limbic, 2023). Integrates with existing NHS systems in many trusts.

Limitations: Black box algorithm—difficult to understand why it makes specific recommendations. Limited transparency about training data and potential biases. Should inform clinical decisions, not replace them. Some patients find automated assessment impersonal.

When to use: Service-level implementation for initial triage rather than individual prescription. Helpful for managing high volumes of referrals. Essential to maintain human oversight and not treat algorithmic suggestions as definitive.

3.4 Beyond Wellness Apps

Here's what distinguishes **digital therapeutics** from the thousands of mental health apps flooding the market: evidence, regulation, and accountability.

Wellness apps track mood, offer meditation, provide inspirational quotes, and teach breathing exercises. Most are free or cheap. Many are helpful to some degree. But they're not medical interventions. They don't have evidence from rigorous trials. They're not regulated. Nobody is legally accountable if they don't work or cause harm.

Digital therapeutics undergo clinical trials, receive regulatory approval as medical devices, make specific therapeutic claims based on evidence, and create accountability for outcomes (Digital Therapeutics Alliance, 2021). When you prescribe DTx, you're taking on clinical responsibility similar to prescribing medication.

This matters for several reasons:

Professional liability: If you recommend a wellness app and it doesn't help, that's unfortunate but not negligence. If you prescribe a digital therapeutic that's contraindicated or used inappropriately, you could face professional consequences. The Nursing and Midwifery Council increasingly addresses technology use in practice standards (NMC, 2023).

Patient expectations: Saying "this app might help" is different from "I'm prescribing this digital treatment." The latter creates expectation of efficacy, need for monitoring, and accountability for outcomes. Patients reasonably expect prescribed treatments to be evidence-based.

Insurance and commissioning: NHS England and CCGs commission digital therapeutics in some areas, meaning they're free to patients when prescribed appropriately. Wellness apps are out-of-pocket. The distinction affects access equity.

Data protection: Regulated digital therapeutics must comply with UK GDPR, NHS data standards, and clinical governance requirements (ICO, 2018). Random wellness apps often have appalling privacy practices—selling data, inadequate security, unclear terms. When you recommend something, you're implicitly vouching for its safety, including data safety.

The grey zone: Some apps blur boundaries. Headspace offers meditation that's evidence-informed but not DTx-level evidence. Big White Wall provides peer support that's helpful but not therapeutic in medical sense. Moodpath tracks symptoms well but offers limited intervention. These can be valuable but shouldn't be presented as primary treatment.

3.5 Funding and Access

This is where idealism meets NHS reality. Evidence-based digital therapeutics exist. Patients might benefit. But who pays, and who gets access?

NHS commissioning of digital mental health tools is fragmented. Some CCGs fund specific platforms. Others don't. Even within regions, access varies by GP practice. You might work in a trust where Sleepio is freely available on prescription, while the trust 20 miles away offers nothing (NHS England, 2023).

IAPT services increasingly incorporate digital options, particularly for stepped care models. Someone with mild anxiety might receive digital CBT before waitlisting for face-to-face therapy. This is cost-effective and evidence-based, but also raises concerns about digital solutions being used primarily to manage demand rather than improve outcomes (Brabyn et al., 2016).

Patient self-funding is common for better platforms. Sleepio costs around £50 for full program. Deprexis is similar. That's cheap compared to private therapy but significant for people on benefits or tight budgets. You're creating a two-tier system if you prescribe things patients must buy themselves.

Free tiers exist for platforms like Wysa and Headspace, but functionality is limited. The evidence-based content often sits behind paywalls. You end up recommending half-measures because full interventions aren't accessible.

Equity implications are enormous. Digital therapeutics require smartphones, data plans, technological literacy, and time to engage with programs. They implicitly favor younger, more educated, more affluent populations (Torous et al., 2020). If digital tools become primary provision for common mental health problems, you risk widening health inequalities rather than closing them.

Some trusts addressed this by providing devices and data plans to patients who need them, but that's exceptional rather than standard. Most places assume everyone has necessary technology and skills. That assumption is wrong and harmful.

Social prescribing might offer a model. Just as you can prescribe gym memberships or art classes in some areas through social prescribing pathways, digital therapeutics could be integrated similarly—funded through non-clinical budgets with clear access criteria (Chatterjee et al., 2018).

The current reality? You need to know what's available in your specific area, which platforms your trust has commissioned, and what patients can access without paying. Then you navigate based on individual circumstances, knowing that your recommendations will be constrained by resources as much as evidence.

3.6 What You've Learned

Digital therapeutics represent a genuine advancement in mental health treatment delivery. They extend your reach, provide evidence-based interventions between appointments, and offer access to people who might not receive anything otherwise. The evidence for specific conditions—particularly insomnia, anxiety, and mild-to-moderate depression—is solid enough that NICE and NHS England recommend them.

But they're not magic. Effect sizes are modest. Dropout rates are high. They work better with human support than alone. And access is frustratingly unequal, with availability depending more on geography and personal finances than clinical need.

Your role is knowing what exists, understanding the evidence, prescribing appropriately, monitoring outcomes, and advocating for better access. Digital therapeutics should supplement mental health nursing, not substitute for it.

The following chapters explore how to integrate these tools into actual workflow—having conversations with patients about digital interventions, monitoring engagement, and using DTx data to inform face-to-face sessions.

Chapter 4.0: Reclaiming Your Time

Picture your typical Tuesday. You arrive at 9 a.m. with eight patients scheduled for face-to-face contact. By noon, you've seen three. The rest of your morning disappeared into documentation, urgent emails, system updates that somehow took 40 minutes, and a phone call with a patient in crisis that you then spent another 25 minutes documenting.

You're not inefficient. You're not lazy. You're drowning in administrative tasks that have nothing to do with why you became a mental health nurse. Research shows that community psychiatric nurses spend 40-60% of their time on documentation and administrative work rather than direct patient care (Royal College of Nursing, 2022). That's not a workflow problem—it's a systemic crisis that AI tools might actually help solve.

This chapter isn't about making you work faster. It's about using technology to reclaim time currently wasted on tasks that don't require your clinical expertise, so you can spend more hours doing work that genuinely needs a human being with your training and judgment.

4.1 Documentation That Works

Let's start with the biggest time thief: **clinical documentation**. You know the routine. After every patient contact, you open the electronic health record system, navigate through multiple screens, fill in mandatory fields, write narrative notes capturing mental state examination, risk assessment, interventions provided, and care plan updates. Twenty to thirty minutes per patient, easily. Some trusts report nurses spending more time documenting care than delivering it (Poissant et al., 2005).

Voice-to-text AI tools are the simplest intervention. Instead of typing, you talk. The software converts speech to text in real-time. Modern systems understand medical terminology with reasonable accuracy—they won't turn "anhedonia" into "Anna don't know ya" like your phone's autocorrect might.

Dragon Medical One, widely deployed in NHS trusts, achieves 99% accuracy for medical vocabulary after brief training on your voice patterns (Nuance, 2023). You can dictate notes immediately after appointments, speaking naturally rather than hunting for keys on a keyboard. The time savings are real: studies show voice recognition reduces documentation time by 30-40% compared to typing (Hammana et al., 2015).

Here's what that looks like practically. You finish a session with Marcus, a 28-year-old man with social anxiety (composite example). Instead of sitting at your desk typing, you open the voice documentation app on your phone and speak while walking to your next appointment:

"Mental state examination for Marcus Chen, clinic appointment November 8th 2025. Appearance and behavior: casually dressed, good eye contact today compared to last session, relaxed posture. Speech: normal rate and tone, more spontaneous than previous contacts. Mood subjectively described as 'better, less anxious about work.' Affect: congruent, bright. Thoughts: no suicidal ideation, reduced social anxiety rumination, reports successfully attending team meeting without panic. Perception: no abnormalities. Cognition: intact. Insight: good, understands anxiety patterns. Risk assessment: low current risk..."

The system generates formatted text. You review for accuracy, add any details the algorithm missed, and approve. Five minutes instead of twenty.

Ambient clinical intelligence takes this further. The AI doesn't wait for you to dictate after the session—it listens during the conversation itself and generates documentation automatically

(Quiroz et al., 2019). Systems like Nuance DAX and Microsoft's Healthcare Bot can record clinical encounters, identify relevant information, and produce draft notes.

The technology works through natural language processing algorithms that distinguish clinically significant content from general conversation. If you ask about sleep and the patient describes nighttime waking, the system captures that. If you discuss weekend plans, it (theoretically) ignores it. The algorithm structures information into appropriate documentation sections—presenting complaint, history, mental state examination, plan.

A pilot at Guy's and St Thomas' NHS Foundation Trust tested ambient documentation for mental health assessments (composite example based on industry reports). Nurses wore a recording device during initial assessments. The AI generated draft notes covering presenting problems, symptom history, risk factors, and mental state examination. Nurses reviewed and edited the drafts, typically spending 5-8 minutes on review compared to 25-30 minutes writing notes from scratch.

Patient feedback was mixed. Some appreciated that the nurse maintained eye contact throughout rather than looking at a computer screen. Others felt uncomfortable being recorded, wondering if the AI accurately captured nuance or might misinterpret statements taken out of context. The trust implemented strict protocols: recording only with explicit patient consent, automatic deletion after note generation, and human review of every AI-generated draft before finalizing.

Template automation uses AI to learn your documentation patterns and pre-populate fields. If you always assess mood, sleep, appetite, energy, and concentration when seeing patients with depression, the system creates a template with those prompts. As you complete more documentation, the algorithm identifies your common phrases and offers to auto-complete them.

The danger here is documentation becoming formulaic—every note looking identical because you're just accepting AI suggestions rather than describing this specific patient on this specific day. Research on electronic health records shows template-driven documentation often sacrifices clinical nuance for efficiency (Rosenbloom et al., 2011). You save time but lose the rich narrative that captures what's actually happening.

The balance: use templates for structure, but demand that you write unique content for each patient. The template provides the framework—presenting complaint, history, mental state, risk, plan—but you describe what you observed and discussed. The AI shouldn't write your clinical thinking; it should just handle formatting.

Legal and governance considerations complicate all of this. Under UK law and NMC standards, you remain professionally accountable for all documentation, regardless of how it was generated (NMC, 2023). If an AI tool produces inaccurate notes and you don't catch the error, you're responsible. If voice recognition misinterprets "denies suicidal ideation" as "endorses suicidal ideation" and you fail to notice, that's clinical negligence.

Some content must remain human-generated. Risk assessments, clinical formulations, and care planning require your judgment. AI can structure the documentation, but you must do the thinking. Trust policies vary—some allow AI-assisted documentation for routine contacts but require manual entry for high-risk situations. Know your local guidelines before implementing these tools.

Data governance is equally important. Who has access to voice recordings? How long are they stored? What happens to data used to train AI systems? Your trust's information governance lead needs to approve any AI documentation tool before you use it clinically. GDPR requirements apply—patients must know their data is being processed by AI, understand what that means, and have the right to object (ICO, 2018).

4.2 Scheduling and Triage

AI-powered triage systems are increasingly common in mental health services. As we discussed in Chapter 1.0, platforms like Limbic Access analyze patient responses during initial contact and recommend appropriate care pathways (Limbic, 2023). Some systems review referral information and prioritize based on urgency. Others monitor ongoing patients and flag those needing earlier review.

The technology works by applying machine learning algorithms to historical data showing which patient characteristics predicted which outcomes. Someone with specific symptom patterns, risk factors, and demographic features gets categorized as needing urgent, routine, or low-intensity intervention based on what happened to similar patients previously (Chekroud et al., 2021).

Here's the critical question: when do you override the algorithm? The system flags Aisha, a 42-year-old woman with recurrent depression (composite example), as routine priority. The algorithm notes stable symptoms over recent months, good medication adherence, strong social support, and no recent crisis. It recommends scheduling her within standard timeframes—probably three to four weeks.

But you read the referral properly. You notice that while her depression symptoms are stable, she mentions her elderly mother just received a terminal cancer diagnosis. You know from experience that anticipated bereavement is a significant stressor that might not show up in depression severity scores yet. You override the algorithm and schedule her within a week.

That's appropriate clinical judgment. The AI spotted patterns in structured data. You spotted context in narrative information. Both matter. The risk is trusting algorithms so completely that you stop reading referrals thoroughly, assuming the machine caught everything important. It didn't (Rudin, 2019).

Evidence on AI triage effectiveness is mixed. A 2021 study comparing algorithmic triage to human triage in mental health services found similar outcomes for most patients, with AI slightly better at identifying low-risk cases who could be managed in primary care and slightly worse at detecting subtle indicators of domestic violence or trauma that weren't explicitly stated (Graham et al., 2021). The algorithm processed referrals faster and more consistently, but missed nuance that experienced nurses caught.

Predictive scheduling uses AI to anticipate high-demand periods and adjust capacity proactively. The system analyzes historical patterns—when do crisis contacts spike? When do patients most frequently miss appointments? When do referrals increase?—and forecasts future demand (Batal et al., 2001).

A mental health trust in Manchester (composite example) implemented predictive scheduling for their crisis team. The algorithm identified patterns: crisis contacts increased significantly on Monday mornings, likely reflecting weekend deteriorations. Contacts spiked during January and early February, consistent with research on seasonal mood patterns. Demand surged immediately after local news coverage of suicide deaths.

The trust adjusted staffing based on predictions, ensuring more nurses on duty during high-risk periods and using quieter times for training or administrative catch-up. They reduced wait times for crisis assessment by 35% and decreased staff overtime by 20% (Batal et al., 2001). The AI didn't create more resources—it just distributed existing capacity more intelligently.

The limitations: predictive algorithms struggle with genuinely unexpected events. A local factory closure causing mass unemployment, a severe weather event disrupting community services, a celebrity suicide prompting copycat ideation—these aren't predictable from historical patterns. You still need human oversight recognizing when circumstances have changed in ways the algorithm can't foresee.

Automating appointment reminders seems straightforward until you think about the human element. SMS reminders reduce missed appointments by about 30% compared to no reminders (Car et al., 2012). Automated phone calls add another 10-15%. The technology works and saves enormous amounts of administrative time.

But there's a balance between efficiency and warmth. A text message saying "You have an appointment with your mental health nurse tomorrow at 2 p.m." conveys information. A message saying "Hi James, looking forward to seeing you tomorrow at 2 p.m. for our chat. Reply if you need to reschedule" feels more personal. The first takes zero staff time. The second requires someone to write personalized messages for each patient—exactly what you're trying to avoid.

Some trusts use AI to generate personalized-seeming messages that aren't actually personalized. The algorithm inserts the patient's first name, references their last appointment date, and uses varied phrasing so messages don't all sound identical. Patients receive something that feels individual without anyone manually writing it.

The ethical question: are you misleading patients by creating an illusion of personal attention that doesn't exist? Research on patient attitudes toward AI communication shows mixed results—some people don't mind automation as long as services are accessible, while others feel devalued by algorithmic interactions (Laranjo et al., 2018). There's no universal answer, but patients deserve honesty about what's human and what's automated.

Follow-up automation raises similar issues. After discharge from crisis care, patients might receive automated check-in messages at one week, two weeks, and one month. If they respond indicating problems, the message gets flagged for human review. If they don't respond at all after several attempts, someone follows up personally.

This can genuinely improve outcomes by catching deterioration early. A study in New Zealand implemented automated text follow-ups for people discharged after mental health crisis (Furber et al.,

2020). Readmission rates dropped by 12% compared to standard care, likely because the system identified people struggling before full relapse occurred. Patients reported feeling supported by regular contact, even though they knew it was automated.

The risk is that automated follow-up replaces human contact entirely rather than supplementing it. If follow-up becomes just algorithmic check-ins without any personal phone calls or appointments, you've lost something important. The technology should enhance care, not substitute for it.

4.3 Your AI Workflow

Let's get concrete about time savings. Here's what a typical workday looks like before and after implementing AI tools effectively:

Before AI integration:

- 9:00 - 9:30: Arrive, check emails (18 messages overnight, 3 urgent), review patient list for day
- 9:30 - 10:30: First appointment with patient experiencing depression
- 10:30 - 11:00: Document previous appointment (type comprehensive notes, update care plan, send communication to GP)
- 11:00 - 12:00: Second appointment with patient in early recovery from psychosis
- 12:00 - 12:30: Document second appointment
- 12:30 - 1:00: Lunch (actually spent responding to urgent emails and checking on a patient who missed appointment)
- 1:00 - 2:00: Third appointment
- 2:00 - 2:30: Document third appointment
- 2:30 - 3:30: MDT meeting discussing complex cases
- 3:30 - 4:00: Attempt to catch up on referrals, realize you're behind on care plan reviews
- 4:00 - 5:00: Fourth appointment (late start because previous tasks ran over)

- 5:00 - 5:45: Document fourth appointment, realize you haven't completed mandatory training module due this week
- 5:45 - 6:15: Stay late finishing documentation and administrative tasks

Result: Four patient contacts, 90 minutes of direct clinical time consumed by documentation, chronic feeling of being behind, working through lunch, staying late.

After AI integration:

- 9:00 - 9:30: Arrive, AI system has flagged 3 urgent emails and deprioritized routine messages, review patient list with AI-generated summaries of relevant recent history
- 9:30 - 10:30: First appointment, voice dictation captures notes in real-time
- 10:30 - 10:40: Review and approve AI-generated documentation, send automated communication to GP using template
- 10:40 - 11:40: Second appointment, ambient AI records and drafts notes
- 11:40 - 11:50: Review AI-generated documentation, add clinical formulation and care plan updates
- 11:50 - 12:50: Third appointment
- 12:50 - 1:00: Dictate notes using voice recognition
- 1:00 - 1:30: Actual lunch break
- 1:30 - 2:00: Fourth appointment (started early because you're not behind)
- 2:00 - 2:10: Review and approve documentation
- 2:10 - 3:10: Fifth appointment (yes, you're seeing an additional patient because you have time)
- 3:10 - 3:20: Documentation
- 3:20 - 4:00: MDT meeting
- 4:00 - 5:00: Catch up on referrals, complete three care plan reviews that were pending, actually do mandatory training module
- 5:00: Leave on time

Result: Five patient contacts (25% increase), documentation time reduced from 90 minutes to 40 minutes, lunch break taken, left on time, completed administrative tasks during working hours.

That's the realistic potential. Not magic, not doubling your productivity, but reclaiming maybe 15-20% of your time currently lost to inefficient processes (Topol, 2019). Over a month, that's multiple hours that could be patient contact, professional development, or—radical thought—not working late.

Realistic expectations matter here. AI won't eliminate administrative burden. Some documentation will always require human input—complex clinical formulations, care planning, risk management decisions. You still need to check emails personally, have difficult conversations with families, attend meetings, and do the thousand small tasks that keep services running.

AI also creates some new work. You need to review AI-generated documentation for accuracy. You need to catch algorithmic errors. You need to override inappropriate triage decisions. Implementing new systems requires training time upfront. Not all AI tools work smoothly—some are clunky, crash frequently, or create as many problems as they solve.

But the time audit doesn't lie. Track your actual time for a week. How many hours do you spend on tasks that genuinely require your clinical expertise? How many hours go to formatting documents, scheduling appointments, chasing referrals, completing mandatory fields in systems that could auto-populate? The latter is where AI can help.

Creating your AI efficiency protocol means identifying which tools address your actual workflow bottlenecks. If documentation is your main time thief, prioritize voice recognition or ambient AI. If triage consumes hours, focus on algorithmic support there. If you're constantly scheduling and rescheduling appointments, automated reminders and predictive capacity management might help most.

Start small. Pick one tool, implement it properly, evaluate whether it genuinely saves time, then expand if it works. Don't implement five AI systems simultaneously and expect smooth integration. That's a recipe for chaos, technical problems, and staff resistance.

Track metrics. How much time are you saving? Are you seeing more patients? Is documentation quality maintained? Are you leaving work on time more often? If the answer to most of these is yes, you're implementing AI effectively. If not, you might be using technology for technology's sake rather than solving real problems.

4.4 Moving Forward Efficiently

The goal isn't maximum efficiency—it's sustainable practice. AI tools should help you provide better care without burning out, see patients who need you without sacrificing documentation quality, and go home on time without feeling guilty about uncompleted work.

Some of you will have access to sophisticated AI systems funded by your trusts. Others will be working with minimal technology, doing your best with inadequate resources. The principles apply regardless: use whatever tools you have to protect your time for work that genuinely needs human expertise, automate what doesn't, and maintain clinical judgment throughout.

Technology alone won't solve workforce crises, inadequate funding, or impossible caseloads. But it might give you back enough time to remember why you chose this profession in the first place—because you're good at helping people, and you care about doing it well.

Chapter 5.0: AI Enhanced Diagnostics

Your patient sits across from you describing symptoms that could indicate major depression, adjustment disorder, hypothyroidism, early dementia, or substance withdrawal. You're weighing possibilities based on pattern recognition developed over years of practice. Meanwhile, an algorithm running in the background has processed 50,000 similar presentations and calculated the probability of each diagnosis based on symptom clusters, demographic factors, and medical history.

Who's right? Sometimes you. Sometimes the machine. Ideally, both—because the best diagnostic accuracy comes from combining algorithmic pattern recognition with human clinical judgment (Topol, 2019). This chapter teaches you how to interpret AI-generated risk scores, integrate diagnostic support systems into your assessments, and know when to trust the algorithm versus when to override it completely.

5.1 Interpreting Risk Scores

AI risk calculators are becoming standard in mental health services. You open a patient's record and see scores: suicide risk 67%, relapse probability 42%, crisis likelihood within 14 days 28%. What do these numbers actually mean, and what should you do with them?

The algorithms work by analyzing multiple data points—age, diagnosis, previous admissions, medication adherence, recent life events, documented symptoms, communication patterns—and comparing them to historical datasets showing which combinations predicted which outcomes (Belsher et al., 2019). If 67 out of 100 previous patients with this profile attempted suicide, the current patient gets flagged at 67% risk.

That sounds scientific. It's actually deeply problematic for several reasons. First, risk isn't static—it changes hour by hour based on factors algorithms can't measure, like an argument with a partner or sudden job loss. Second, the base rate matters enormously. If suicide attempts occur in 1% of your patient population, even a highly accurate algorithm will generate far more false positives than true positives (Large et al., 2011). Third, algorithms trained on one population often perform poorly on different populations, raising concerns about bias and equity.

Here's what the numbers mean practically. A 67% suicide risk score doesn't mean this person has a 67% chance of attempting suicide. It means they share characteristics with a group where 67% attempted in the dataset used to train the algorithm. Their actual risk might be 90% or 10% depending on factors the algorithm didn't capture.

The traffic light system simplifies risk into categories that feel more actionable: green (low risk), amber (moderate risk), red (high risk). This is how many NHS trusts present algorithmic risk scores. The benefit is clarity—staff know immediately which patients need urgent attention. The danger is oversimplification—treating everyone in the amber category identically when their actual circumstances vary enormously.

Let's work through an example. You're reviewing your caseload, and the system flags three patients as amber risk:

Patient 1: Diego, 52-year-old man with bipolar disorder. Recent score of 58% based on medication non-adherence, reduced appointment attendance, and increased crisis line contacts. You call him. He's been struggling to afford prescriptions due to job loss but is now receiving benefits and plans to collect medication today. He's stressed but stable, with good insight. The elevated risk score reflected a temporary financial crisis that's resolving.

Patient 2: Priya, 34-year-old woman with recurrent depression. Score of 51% based on increased symptoms documented at last appointment. You call her. She reports worsening mood, increased suicidal ideation (though no plan), and hopelessness about her situation. She's appropriate for amber category and needs escalated care—earlier appointment, increased contact frequency, medication review.

Patient 3: Li, 29-year-old non-binary person with anxiety and trauma history. Score of 63% primarily based on demographic factors (age, diagnosis) rather than current presentation. You review recent contacts—Li has been engaging well, practicing coping skills, making progress in trauma therapy. The algorithm flagged them because people with their characteristics sometimes deteriorate rapidly, but Li is actually doing well. This is a false positive requiring no action beyond routine follow-up.

Same amber category, three entirely different clinical scenarios requiring different responses. The algorithm provided a starting point for prioritization—it prompted you to review these three patients rather than others. But your judgment determined appropriate action in each case.

When AI gets it wrong happens frequently enough that you need clear protocols for clinical override. Research on suicide prediction algorithms shows even the best systems miss 30-40% of attempts while flagging many people who never deteriorate (Belsher et al., 2019). That's not grounds for abandoning the technology—your clinical judgment alone misses attempts too—but it's grounds for combining both approaches.

False positives occur when algorithms flag low-risk patients as high-risk. This wastes resources (you're urgently assessing people who don't need it) and potentially causes harm (patients flagged as high-risk when they feel fine might feel invalidated or mistrusted). Some false positives are acceptable if it means catching more true positives, but the ratio matters. If you're doing 20 urgent assessments to catch 2 actual crises, that might be worthwhile. If you're doing 100 to catch 2, you've overwhelmed services and created alert fatigue—staff start ignoring flags because they're usually wrong.

False negatives are more dangerous—algorithms missing high-risk patients who subsequently deteriorate. A study analyzing electronic health records in a large mental health trust found that algorithmic risk prediction missed 35% of patients who attempted suicide within 30 days of assessment (Tran et al., 2014). These weren't random misses. The algorithm struggled particularly with patients whose risk escalated due to sudden life events (relationship breakdown, job loss) rather than gradually worsening mental state.

This is why you can't outsource risk assessment to machines. The algorithm spots patterns in historical data. You spot context in current presentation. Both matter. The patient whose risk score is green but who just told you their relationship ended and they're losing their home needs urgent assessment regardless of what the algorithm says.

Documenting clinical override protects you professionally and improves system performance. If you disagree with an algorithmic risk score, document: (1) what the algorithm recommended, (2) your assessment, (3) clinical reasoning for your decision, (4) actions taken based on your judgment. This creates a clear record showing you considered multiple sources of information and made a reasoned clinical decision.

Documentation like this also helps developers improve algorithms. If you consistently override scores in particular circumstances, that's valuable feedback indicating the algorithm is missing something important. Some systems incorporate override data to refine predictions—if experienced nurses regularly flag false negatives the algorithm missed, the next version can weight those factors differently.

5.2 Diagnostic Support Systems

Symptom checkers are controversial but increasingly common. Patients complete questionnaires describing symptoms, and algorithms suggest possible diagnoses. Some operate like decision trees—if you answer yes to questions A, B, and C, you're guided toward diagnosis X. More sophisticated systems use machine learning to recognize patterns across multiple symptoms simultaneously (Semigran et al., 2015).

The evidence on diagnostic accuracy is mixed. A 2015 study tested 23 symptom checker apps by inputting standardized case vignettes (Semigran et al., 2015). The correct diagnosis appeared in the top 3 suggestions about 50% of the time—better than random chance, worse than human clinicians. Accuracy varied dramatically by condition; algorithms were decent at identifying common conditions like depression but terrible at rare presentations.

In mental health settings, symptom checkers serve different functions than medical diagnosis. You're not using AI to diagnose schizophrenia versus bipolar disorder from a list of symptoms—that requires comprehensive assessment. You're using it to structure initial data collection, ensure you ask about relevant symptom domains, and identify presentations that might need specialist input you hadn't considered.

Elena, a 38-year-old woman, completes a digital symptom assessment before her first appointment (composite example). She reports low mood, poor sleep, concentration difficulties, and fatigue. The algorithm identifies depressive symptoms but also flags questions about racing thoughts, increased energy, and reduced sleep need—screening for bipolar features. You might have assessed for this anyway, but the prompt ensures you don't miss it. The assessment takes pressure off you to remember every screening question while allowing you to focus on rapport-building and therapeutic engagement.

Natural language processing in assessments analyzes how people describe symptoms, not just which symptoms they endorse. Research shows that word choice, sentence structure, and speech patterns contain diagnostic information (Corcoran et al., 2018). People experiencing psychosis use more abstract language and make more tangential connections. People with depression speak more slowly with longer pauses. Manic speech is faster with more tangential shifts.

Some diagnostic systems analyze written or recorded clinical notes to identify linguistic markers of mental illness. A study at Columbia University found that NLP algorithms analyzing clinical interview transcripts predicted psychosis onset up to two years in advance with 80% accuracy by detecting increased thought disorganization in speech patterns (Corcoran et al., 2018).

This feels uncomfortably close to thought policing. We're analyzing not just what people say but how they say it, using deviations from typical speech as indicators of pathology. The ethical implications are significant—particularly given that communication patterns vary by culture, education, and neurodiversity. What looks like disorganized thinking to an algorithm trained on British English speakers might be normal communication in other languages or cultures.

The practical application in your work: NLP systems might flag concerning language patterns in patient communications—crisis messages with hopeless language, emails showing cognitive disorganization, or appointment cancellations with concerning wording. The algorithm draws your attention to something worth exploring. You decide what it means.

Integrating AI with clinical interviews requires balance. You can't conduct proper mental state examination while staring at a computer screen checking algorithmic prompts. But you also can't ignore potentially valuable information just because it came from AI rather than your own observation.

The approach that works: prepare before the appointment by reviewing AI-generated summaries of relevant history, current risk scores, and flagged concerns. During the appointment, focus fully on the patient—maintain eye contact, build rapport, conduct your assessment using clinical skills developed over years. After the appointment, compare your assessment with what AI systems flagged. Did you miss anything? Did the algorithm highlight something you dismissed as insignificant? Was its risk score consistent with your clinical judgment?

This comparative process improves both your practice and algorithmic accuracy. You catch things you might have missed. The system learns from patterns in your overrides. Over time, the integration becomes seamless—AI handles pattern recognition across thousands of data points while you handle nuance, context, and therapeutic relationship.

Real-world scenario: You're conducting a first assessment with Marcus, a 45-year-old man referred for low mood and anxiety (composite example). Before the appointment, you review the AI-generated summary: referral information, relevant medical history, completed questionnaires showing moderate depression and severe anxiety scores, algorithmic risk score of 42% flagged amber.

During the session, you explore his history, current symptoms, life circumstances, and coping strategies. He describes panic attacks triggered by work stress, insomnia, and anhedonia. He also mentions—almost as an aside—that he's recently stopped seeing friends and is drinking more to manage anxiety. You probe further. He's consuming 30-40 units of alcohol weekly, up from 10-15 units six months ago. This wasn't captured in the questionnaires because they asked about typical drinking, not recent changes.

Your clinical assessment concludes he's at higher risk than the 42% score suggested because of escalating alcohol use in response to anxiety—a concerning pattern not apparent in questionnaire responses. You document this clearly, adjust the risk category, and develop a care plan addressing both anxiety and alcohol use. The AI provided a starting point; your interview captured what structured questions missed.

5.3 Collaborative Decision Making

The **"centaur model"** of human-AI collaboration comes from chess. After computers became better than humans at chess, a new form emerged: advanced chess, where human players working with computers outperformed computers alone or humans alone (Kasparov, 2017). The human contributed strategic thinking and pattern recognition; the computer contributed calculation and evaluation of millions of positions. Together, they were stronger than either separately.

Mental health nursing can work similarly. AI contributes pattern recognition across vast datasets—spotting combinations of symptoms, behaviors, and risk factors you might miss. You contribute contextual understanding, therapeutic relationship, ethical reasoning, and judgment about what matters clinically versus what's just data noise (Topol, 2019).

This works when both parties play to their strengths. AI is excellent at identifying patients whose profile matches historical patterns predicting deterioration. You're excellent at recognizing when someone's current circumstances make them atypical despite their profile. AI processes more information than you ever could. You understand human complexity better than any algorithm.

The breakdown occurs when either replaces the other. Pure algorithmic decision-making misses context and humanity. Pure human judgment misses patterns only visible across populations. The combination—AI flagging concerning patterns plus your interpretation of what those patterns mean for this specific person—produces better outcomes than either alone (Cabitza et al., 2017).

Teaching patients about AI-informed care prevents confusion and builds trust. Many people don't realize algorithms are involved in their care. They see risk scores or treatment recommendations without understanding where these came from. Transparency matters both ethically and practically.

Here's how that conversation might go with Aisha, a 31-year-old woman with depression:

You: "I want to explain something about how we monitor your care. Our electronic system uses what's called AI—artificial intelligence—to help identify when someone might be struggling, so we can reach out proactively rather than waiting for you to contact us in crisis."

Aisha: "So a computer is making decisions about my care?"

You: "Not exactly. The computer analyzes patterns—things like how often you're attending appointments, medication collection records, responses to questionnaires, that kind of thing. If it spots patterns that in the past have meant someone was deteriorating, it flags you for me to check in. But I make all the actual clinical decisions. The computer can't know how you're actually doing—only you and I can determine that through conversation."

Aisha: "What information does it use?"

You: "Everything in your clinical record—diagnoses, medications, appointment history, anything documented from our sessions, scores from questionnaires you've completed. It doesn't access anything outside the NHS system, like your social media or personal emails. Everything is protected by the same confidentiality standards as your regular medical records."

Aisha: "Does it ever get it wrong?"

You: "Yes, regularly. Sometimes it flags people as high-risk who are actually fine—we call those false alarms. Sometimes it misses people who are struggling. That's why I don't rely on it alone. It's a tool that helps me prioritize who needs urgent attention, but my clinical assessment of how you're actually doing always takes priority."

This explanation is honest about capabilities and limitations, explains what data is used, and clarifies that humans make final decisions. Patients deserve this information, and most appreciate the transparency.

When to bring AI data into MDT meetings depends on the meeting's purpose and the team's literacy around AI. If you're discussing a complex case and algorithmic risk scores provide useful context—"the system flagged her as high-risk three days before she presented in crisis, which might have given us a window for earlier intervention if we'd had capacity to respond"—that's relevant.

If you're discussing someone the algorithm flagged but your assessment suggests is stable, mention this too: "He's scored amber risk for the past month, but his actual presentation has been consistently good, suggesting the algorithm is picking up historical factors rather than current risk." This helps colleagues understand algorithmic limitations.

What's unhelpful: treating algorithmic scores as definitive truth. Don't say "the AI says she's high-risk" as if that settles the matter. Do say "the system flagged her as high-risk based on these factors, and my assessment confirms concerning deterioration." The former abdicates responsibility; the latter integrates multiple sources of information.

When to leave AI out of MDT discussions: when it adds no useful information beyond what's apparent from clinical presentation, when the team doesn't understand how algorithms work (you'll waste time explaining rather than discussing the patient), or when algorithmic recommendations conflict with clear clinical consensus and mentioning them would just confuse matters.

The goal is using AI to enhance clinical discussions, not to dominate them or replace clinical reasoning. Algorithms provide information. Humans make decisions. Keep that hierarchy clear.

5.4 Essential Takeaways

AI-enhanced diagnostics and risk assessment offer real value when used appropriately: earlier identification of deterioration, more consistent screening, flagging of concerning patterns you might miss in overwhelming caseloads. They're not replacing your clinical judgment—they're augmenting it with pattern recognition at a scale humans can't match.

But they're far from perfect. False positives and false negatives are common. Algorithms trained on one population perform poorly on others. Systems miss context and nuance that you catch immediately. Your professional responsibility is knowing when to trust algorithmic suggestions and when to override them based on clinical judgment.

The future of mental health nursing isn't nurses or AI—it's nurses and AI working together, each contributing what they do best. Your job is learning to be an effective collaborator with these systems while maintaining the human expertise, empathy, and judgment that AI cannot replicate.

Chapter 6.0: Prescribing Digital Therapeutics

You're about to recommend that someone download an app as part of their mental health treatment. This feels different from suggesting they try journaling or practice breathing exercises. Those are general wellness recommendations. This is clinical intervention delivered via software—and you're taking on professional responsibility for the recommendation.

Prescribing digital therapeutics requires different skills than prescribing medication. You need to assess not just clinical appropriateness but also technological literacy, access to devices, motivation for self-directed work, and whether the patient's problems actually match what the app addresses. You need to set realistic expectations about what digital tools can and cannot do. And you need to monitor engagement and outcomes the same way you would any other treatment.

This chapter gives you the practical framework for incorporating DTx into your practice competently and safely. We'll cover the clinical conversation, review specific platforms in detail, explore integration with face-to-face care, and address special populations who may struggle with digital interventions.

6.1 The Prescription Conversation

Let's start with the moment where you introduce the idea. You're sitting with James, a 27-year-old man experiencing moderate depression (composite example). He's been on your caseload for six weeks. Medication is helping somewhat, but he's still struggling. You meet every two weeks, which feels insufficient, but you don't have capacity for weekly sessions and he doesn't meet criteria for intensive support.

How to introduce DTx:

You: "I've been thinking about how we can support you between our appointments. Right now we're seeing each other every two weeks, but depression doesn't pause during the weeks we're not meeting. There's a digital tool—basically a program you access through your phone—that provides CBT techniques you can work through at your own pace. It's called Wysa. It won't replace our sessions, but it could give you structured support on the days we're not meeting."

James: "Like an app? I tried some meditation apps before. They were okay but didn't really help."

You: "This is different from general wellness apps. Wysa is specifically designed for anxiety and depression, with evidence showing it helps reduce symptoms. It uses conversational AI—you type messages describing how you're feeling, and it responds with appropriate techniques. Think of it as homework between our sessions that's a bit more interactive than just worksheets."

James: "Does it cost money?"

You: "There's a free version with core features that should work for what you need. If you wanted the premium version with more content, it's about £60 for three months, but let's start with the free version and see if it's helpful first."

James: "What if I don't use it?"

You: "Then we'll try something else. This only works if you actually engage with it—probably 10-15 minutes a few times a week. If you download it and never open it, we've gained nothing. But if you're willing to give it a proper try for a month, I think you might find it helpful."

This conversation covers key elements: explaining what DTx is, distinguishing it from wellness apps, being honest about costs, acknowledging that engagement is voluntary, and setting realistic expectations about effort required.

Matching tools to patients requires clinical judgment about both the problem and the person. A **decision tree** approach helps:

Is the primary problem:

- Depression → Consider Wysa (mild-moderate), Deprexis (moderate), SilverCloud (guided support available)
- Anxiety → Consider Wysa, Headspace (with caveats about evidence), Sanvello
- Insomnia → Sleepio is first-line (strong evidence base)
- PTSD/Trauma → Limited DTx options; specialist input needed
- Psychosis/Bipolar → Very limited DTx; maintain face-to-face care as primary

Patient characteristics:

- Technologically comfortable? → Any platform appropriate
- Limited tech literacy? → Choose simplest interface (Wysa over Deprexis)
- No smartphone? → May need to provide device or use alternative approaches
- High motivation for self-directed work? → Comprehensive programs like Deprexis work well
- Low motivation? → Brief, interactive tools like Wysa better than lengthy modules
- Strong therapeutic alliance with you? → Can use DTx as homework and discuss in sessions
- New to service? → Build relationship first; introduce DTx later

Setting expectations prevents disappointment and disengagement. People need to understand what digital therapeutics can and cannot do before they start.

Digital therapy CAN:

- Provide structured evidence-based techniques between appointments
- Teach coping skills you can practice at your own pace
- Offer support at times when services aren't available (evenings, weekends)
- Help you track symptoms and identify patterns
- Extend the reach of face-to-face therapy through homework and skill practice

Digital therapy CANNOT:

- Replace human therapeutic relationships
- Respond to crisis situations appropriately (always contact crisis services or emergency numbers in crisis)
- Adapt to complex trauma, personality difficulties, or severe mental illness as effectively as specialist human care
- Understand context, nuance, and individual circumstances the way a person can
- Guarantee improvement (just like any treatment, it helps some people a lot, others less so)

Research on patient expectations shows that people who understand DTx as supplementary to human care have better outcomes than those who view it as a substitute (Musiat et al., 2014). Managing expectations upfront improves engagement and satisfaction.

Monitoring engagement means tracking whether people actually use what you prescribed. Most DTx platforms provide clinician dashboards showing user activity—how often they logged in, which modules they completed, symptom scores from app-based questionnaires. This data is clinically useful if you use it to inform conversations rather than judge compliance.

At your next appointment with James, you might say: "I can see you've been using Wysa quite regularly—looks like you logged in five times this week. How has that been going? Have you found any of the techniques helpful?" That's using engagement data to open dialogue about what's working.

If James hadn't engaged at all, the conversation shifts: "I notice Wysa hasn't been opened since we set it up. What got in the way? Was it technical problems, not finding it helpful, or just forgetting about it?" This identifies barriers rather than criticizing.

Therapeutic alliance with digital tools is real but different from human relationship. Research shows people can form attachment to AI chatbots, describe them as supportive, and prefer them over human therapists in certain situations—particularly when discussing embarrassing topics (Lucas et al., 2014). But digital relationships lack reciprocity, genuine empathy, and the kind of attunement that happens between two human beings.

Your job is helping patients use DTx effectively without expecting it to replace human connection. The app provides techniques and structure. You provide empathy, clinical judgment, and genuine care about their wellbeing. Both matter; neither fully substitutes for the other.

6.2 Platform Deep Dive

Let's examine the platforms you're most likely to encounter in detail—not just what they claim but what the evidence shows and when they're clinically appropriate.

Wysa: The Empathetic Chatbot

What it is: Conversational AI delivering CBT techniques, mindfulness exercises, and emotional support through text-based chat. Users type messages describing mood or problems; Wysa responds with validation, questions, and technique suggestions.

Evidence base: Several studies show modest improvements in anxiety and depression symptoms. A 2018 study of 129 users found significant reductions in depression scores over four weeks (Inkster et al., 2018). Effect sizes were small to moderate (d = 0.35-0.44), meaning clinically noticeable but not dramatic improvement. Crucially, outcomes were better for people who engaged regularly—using Wysa at least three times weekly—compared to sporadic users.

Strengths:

- Highly accessible—available 24/7 including evenings and weekends when crisis support is limited
- Conversational interface feels less clinical than working through CBT modules
- Free tier includes substantial content (though premium features require payment)
- Particularly appeals to young adults comfortable with messaging interfaces
- Can complement face-to-face therapy effectively as between-session support
- Provides immediate (albeit algorithmic) response when someone is distressed

Limitations:

- Fully automated with no human oversight unless you pay for premium coaching
- Conversations can feel repetitive after extended use—the AI has limited ability to personalize
- Struggles with complex presentations or situations outside programmed responses
- Sometimes misinterprets input, offering inappropriate suggestions
- Not suitable for crisis despite marketing suggesting 24/7 support (redirects to crisis numbers but can't provide actual crisis intervention)
- Limited evidence for severe depression or anxiety

When to prescribe: Mild-to-moderate anxiety or depression in adults comfortable with technology, as adjunct to face-to-face care or for people on waiting lists. Good for young people who prefer digital communication. Not appropriate as sole treatment for severe symptoms or people in crisis.

Clinical pearl: Frame it explicitly as homework between sessions. Ask patients to try specific Wysa techniques (e.g., thought challenging, breathing exercises) and discuss their experience in your next appointment. This integration makes it feel like part of therapy rather than separate.

Sleepio: Gold Standard Digital CBT-I

What it is: Six-week program delivering cognitive-behavioral therapy for insomnia through animated virtual therapist. Covers sleep restriction, stimulus control, cognitive techniques, relaxation, and sleep hygiene.

Evidence base: Multiple large RCTs showing robust improvements in sleep quality and duration (Espie et al., 2019). Effect sizes comparable to face-to-face CBT-I ($d = 0.87$ for sleep quality). Benefits persist at six-month follow-up. NICE explicitly recommends digital CBT-I as first-line treatment before medication.

Strengths:

- Strong evidence base—probably the best-researched DTx in mental health
- Delivers same content as face-to-face CBT-I, which is treatment of choice for insomnia
- More accessible than face-to-face sleep clinics with long waiting lists
- Cost-effective—cheaper than both sleep medication long-term and therapist-delivered CBT-I
- Engaging interface with good user retention
- Available on NHS prescription in some areas (check local commissioning)

Limitations:

- Requires commitment to sleep restriction protocol, which many find difficult initially
- Takes several weeks to see improvement—not suitable for someone needing immediate help
- Less effective if insomnia is secondary to untreated mental illness (needs to address underlying condition)
- Not suitable for sleep disorders other than insomnia (e.g., sleep apnea, restless leg syndrome)
- Can initially worsen fatigue during sleep restriction phase

When to prescribe: Primary insomnia or insomnia comorbid with stable mental health conditions. Patients need to be motivated enough to complete sleep diaries and follow protocols. Use before prescribing hypnotics. Excellent for people who prefer self-directed treatment or lack access to sleep specialists.

When NOT to prescribe: Acute crisis situations, severe untreated depression or anxiety (treat those first), suspected sleep apnea or other medical sleep disorders (refer for assessment), people unable to commit to structured program.

Clinical pearl: Warn patients upfront that sleep restriction temporarily increases tiredness before improving sleep. Frame this as normal and necessary rather than the program failing. Check in after week one to support adherence through difficult initial phase.

Deprexis: Comprehensive Digital CBT

What it is: Ten interactive modules covering behavioral activation, cognitive restructuring, mindfulness, interpersonal skills, problem-solving, relaxation, and relapse prevention for depression. Users work through at own pace with automated feedback.

Evidence base: Multiple RCTs showing significant depression reduction (Berger et al., 2011). Effect sizes around 0.60-0.80 for guided programs (with therapist support) and 0.30-0.50 for unguided. More effective than waitlist but less effective than face-to-face therapy. Outcomes improve when combined with brief human contact.

Strengths:

- Comprehensive content covering multiple CBT approaches
- Can be used independently or alongside therapy
- Evidence base from multiple trials across different populations
- Allows personalization—users can focus on most relevant modules
- Good for people who've had CBT before and need refresher or maintenance
- Can track progress through built-in outcome measures

Limitations:

- Module-based format feels like online coursework rather than therapy
- Completion rates modest—many start but don't finish
- Less engaging than conversational interfaces like Wysa
- Requires significant motivation for self-directed work
- Works better with therapist guidance than as standalone treatment
- Expensive for self-pay (£50-70 for full program)

When to prescribe: Moderate depression in people who prefer structured, educational approach. Works particularly well when you guide patients through modules and discuss content in sessions. Good for people who previously responded to CBT and want maintenance support. Suitable for those willing to commit to substantial homework.

When NOT to prescribe: Severe depression needing intensive support, people with limited motivation for self-directed work (they won't complete it), crisis situations, patients who find educational approaches unhelpful or patronizing.

Clinical pearl: Don't just prescribe and hope patients complete it independently. Select specific modules relevant to their presentation, assign them as homework, and review content together. This "blended care" approach produces much better outcomes than unguided use.

Limbic Access: AI Triage at Scale

What it is: Not a patient-facing therapeutic tool but a service-level triage system. Analyzes patient responses during initial contact and recommends appropriate care pathways. Used by IAPT services and mental health trusts to route referrals efficiently.

Evidence base: Limited published research but industry data from 100+ NHS services using it (Limbic, 2023). Claims to reduce waiting times and improve triage consistency compared to human-only triage. No peer-reviewed studies comparing outcomes to standard care.

CPN perspective: You're more likely to encounter this as part of service infrastructure than something you prescribe individually. The algorithm routes patients before they reach you, potentially affecting who appears on your caseload and when.

Strengths from nursing perspective:

- Reduces administrative burden of initial triage
- More consistent than human triage (doesn't have bad days or bias from previous case)
- Can handle high referral volumes without additional staff
- Flags high-risk cases for urgent human review
- Potentially reduces waiting times by routing patients efficiently

Concerns from nursing perspective:

- Black box algorithm—difficult to understand why specific recommendations made

- May perpetuate biases in training data
- Risk of deskilling—junior staff don't learn triage judgment
- Patients may find automated assessment impersonal during vulnerable moment of seeking help
- Limited ability to capture nuance in narrative referrals
- Over-reliance could mean human oversight is inadequate

Critical point: Algorithmic triage should supplement human judgment, not replace it. High-risk flags require immediate human review. Routine categorization shouldn't mean no human ever looks at the referral. Patients deserve the option to speak with a person if automated assessment feels insufficient.

Mindfulness and Meditation Apps: Evidence vs Hype

The marketplace is flooded with mindfulness apps making varying claims. Let's separate evidence-based tools from wellness fluff.

Evidence-based:

- **Headspace:** Some research showing anxiety and depression reduction (Flett et al., 2019), though effect sizes are modest and shorter-term than clinical interventions
- **Calm:** Emerging evidence for stress reduction, though most studies are small
- **Insight Timer:** Good range of guided meditations though limited outcome research

Wellness fluff:

- Most apps making claims about curing depression, eliminating anxiety, or transforming mental health have zero evidence
- Generic relaxation or positive thinking apps are not therapeutic interventions
- "Mindfulness" has become marketing term applied to products with no grounding in mindfulness-based stress reduction or mindfulness-based cognitive therapy protocols

Clinical guidance: Mindfulness apps can supplement care for mild anxiety or stress, but shouldn't be confused with evidence-based digital therapeutics. Don't prescribe them as primary treatment. They're helpful adjuncts—like recommending someone take walks for physical health. Useful, generally positive, but not clinical intervention.

6.3 Blended Care Integration

The blended care model combines face-to-face sessions with digital work between appointments. Research consistently shows this produces better outcomes than either approach alone (Erbe et al., 2017). The structure looks like:

Face-to-face session: Assess current state, identify priority issues, teach new skills or techniques, discuss progress and challenges, assign digital homework

Between sessions: Patient uses DTx to practice skills, complete exercises, track symptoms, try techniques in real situations

Next face-to-face session: Review digital work, discuss what was helpful or difficult, refine approach based on patient's experience, assign next round of digital homework

This creates continuity of care that weekly or fortnightly appointments alone can't achieve. The therapeutic work continues between sessions rather than pausing until you meet again.

Using app data clinically requires accessing clinician dashboards most DTx platforms provide. You see engagement metrics (how often did they log in?), completed modules, symptom tracking data, and sometimes content of exercises completed.

Here's how to use this productively with Priya, a 40-year-old woman with anxiety (composite example). You review her Wysa activity before your appointment. She's logged in regularly but engagement dropped sharply this week. In session:

You: "I noticed you were using Wysa pretty consistently, but engagement dropped off in the last few days. What happened?"

Priya: "I just got overwhelmed. Work was chaotic, and I couldn't face doing more things on my to-do list."

You: "That makes sense. When you're overwhelmed, adding tasks—even helpful ones—feels impossible. Let's think about how to make digital tools feel like support rather than pressure. Would it help if we lowered expectations? Maybe just opening Wysa once when you're feeling stressed rather than trying to complete whole exercises?"

This conversation uses engagement data as a springboard for understanding barriers. You're not judging non-compliance; you're exploring what got in the way and problem-solving together.

Troubleshooting low engagement requires distinguishing between three scenarios:

1. Patient issue: Poor motivation, ambivalence about change, overwhelming life circumstances making self-directed work unrealistic

2. App issue: Interface confusing, content not relevant to patient's actual problems, technical glitches, required exercises feel unhelpful or patronizing

3. Prescription issue: You recommended wrong tool for this person, didn't explain clearly what to do, set unrealistic expectations about time commitment

Your assessment determines the response. If it's patient motivation, explore ambivalence and consider whether DTx is appropriate right now. If it's the app, try a different platform or abandon digital approaches. If it's prescription error, acknowledge it and adjust.

Don't blame patients for not engaging. Most non-adherence reflects problems with treatment fit or presentation rather than patient failure (Waller, 2009).

Deprescribing digital tools is as important as prescribing them. If someone's been using a DTx for months with no benefit, continuing is pointless. If they've improved and no longer need support, celebrating success and discontinuing makes sense. If they find it unhelpful or burdensome, forcing continued use damages therapeutic relationship.

Signs it's time to stop:

- No symptom improvement after 8-12 weeks of consistent engagement
- Patient reports DTx unhelpful or makes them feel worse
- Engagement dropped to zero despite problem-solving barriers
- Clinical situation changed (e.g., deteriorated to severity needing intensive support)
- Patient no longer has access to necessary technology
- They've completed program and benefited—job done

Frame discontinuation positively: "We gave Sleepio a good try over two months. Your sleep has improved significantly, so let's stop the structured program and just maintain the habits you've developed. If sleep becomes a problem again, we know this approach works for you."

6.4 Special Populations

Older adults present specific challenges with DTx. Digital literacy varies enormously. Some 70-year-olds navigate technology better than some 30-year-olds, but as a group, older adults have less experience with smartphones and apps (Seifert et al., 2021).

Design matters. Apps with small text, complex navigation, or assumptions about tech familiarity create barriers. Sleepio works reasonably well for older adults because the interface is straightforward. Wysa's messaging format is intuitive for anyone who texts. Deprexis's module structure can feel overwhelming.

Physical limitations matter too. Arthritis makes touch-screen interaction difficult. Vision problems make small screens challenging even with enlarged text. Hearing issues affect apps using audio instructions.

The clinical conversation with older adults needs extra care. Don't assume DTx is inappropriate just because someone is 75. But don't assume they'll figure it out independently either. Offer to walk through setup together. Provide written instructions. Involve family if appropriate and patient consents. Check in more frequently initially to troubleshoot technical problems.

Severe and enduring mental illness is where DTx evidence gets really thin. Most research studies excluded people with psychosis, bipolar disorder, or complex presentations. We have minimal data on whether these tools help, harm, or do nothing for people with severe conditions.

Some limited evidence suggests adjunctive benefits—people with stable schizophrenia using symptom-tracking apps showed modest improvement in self-management (Firth et al., 2017). But this is far from recommending DTx as primary treatment.

Your clinical judgment guides this. Someone with stable bipolar disorder experiencing breakthrough depressive symptoms might benefit from Wysa while you adjust medication. Someone experiencing active psychosis needs intensive human support, not an app. Someone with severe depression and suicidal ideation needs assessment and crisis intervention, not digital CBT modules.

Use DTx for this population only as supplements to comprehensive care, never as substitutes. Monitor closely for deterioration. Be prepared to discontinue if problems worsen or app proves unhelpful.

Cultural considerations are largely unaddressed in current DTx. Most platforms were developed in Western, English-speaking contexts with limited consideration of cultural diversity. The algorithms don't understand cultural variations in symptom expression, help-seeking, or therapeutic approaches (Torous et al., 2020).

Examples of cultural blind spots:

- CBT emphasis on individual autonomy and cognitive restructuring may not align with collectivist cultures valuing family interdependence
- Expression of distress varies culturally—DTx trained on Western presentations may misinterpret symptoms from other cultural contexts
- Therapeutic relationship expectations differ—some cultures expect more directive guidance than app-based self-help provides
- Language matters beyond translation—idioms, metaphors, and communication styles vary

When prescribing DTx to patients from diverse backgrounds, have explicit conversations about cultural fit. Ask: "Does this approach make sense given your background and beliefs? Does the way the app suggests handling problems align with how your family or community typically addresses difficulties?" If not, DTx may be inappropriate or need careful framing.

Digital exclusion is the hardest problem. Not everyone owns a smartphone. Not everyone has reliable internet. Not everyone can afford data plans. If DTx becomes standard care and you lack alternatives for digitally excluded patients, you're creating a two-tier system based on economic access to technology (Torous et al., 2020).

Some trusts addressed this by providing devices and data plans to patients who need them. This is expensive but ethical. Others maintain non-digital alternatives—paper-based CBT workbooks, telephone support, face-to-face provision—ensuring access isn't dependent on technology ownership.

Your role: advocate for patients who can't access digital tools. Don't treat DTx as the only option. Push back if service models assume everyone has smartphones and data. Document when digital exclusion limits care options. Build the case for equitable alternatives.

6.5 Core Insights

Digital therapeutics expand your treatment options when used thoughtfully. They extend your reach without extending your hours, provide structure between appointments, and offer evidence-based interventions to people who otherwise might receive nothing while waiting for services.

But they're not appropriate for everyone, not effective for everything, and never a substitute for human expertise and compassion. Your job is matching the right tool to the right patient at the right time, supporting engagement, monitoring outcomes, and adjusting when approaches aren't working.

DTx are tools in your toolkit—powerful when used appropriately, problematic when overapplied or relied upon excessively. Master their use, but never let technology replace the therapeutic relationship that remains central to effective mental health nursing.

Chapter 7.0: Real World Implementation

Theory is clean. Practice is messy. AI tools that look brilliant in pilot studies often stumble when deployed in actual clinical settings with real patients, overworked staff, and systems that crash on Tuesday mornings because someone updated the wrong server.

This chapter presents case studies from mental health services that implemented AI tools—what succeeded, what failed spectacularly, and what they learned. These aren't hypothetical scenarios. They're composite examples drawn from real implementations across NHS trusts, with identifying details changed but core lessons intact. Your service will make some of these same mistakes. Learning from others' experiences might help you avoid the worst ones.

7.1 AI Risk Screening Integration

The Setting: A community mental health team serving a diverse urban population of about 80,000 people. Caseload per nurse averaged 35-40 patients. Staff were experienced but stretched thin. The trust purchased an AI risk screening system promising to identify patients at elevated risk of crisis or suicide, allowing proactive intervention before deterioration.

What They Tried: The algorithm analyzed electronic health records continuously, flagging patients whose profiles matched historical patterns predicting adverse events. Risk scores updated weekly. Nurses received automated alerts when patients moved from green to amber or amber to red. The system claimed 75% accuracy in predicting crisis within 30 days.

Initial Problems:

The alert volume was overwhelming. In the first month, the system flagged 180 patients across the team—about 45% of the total caseload. Nurses couldn't possibly follow up with everyone urgently. The algorithm was technically working (it caught most people who deteriorated) but generated so many false positives that staff couldn't distinguish signal from noise (Belsher et al., 2019).

The team tried triaging alerts by urgency. Red flags required same-day contact. Amber flags required contact within a week. But "contact" became checking boxes rather than meaningful intervention. A five-minute phone call asking "are you okay?" satisfied the requirement but provided minimal clinical benefit. Staff felt they were serving the algorithm rather than patients.

Trust in the system eroded quickly. When nurses investigated amber flags, they often found patients who were genuinely stable—the algorithm had picked up historical risk factors that weren't currently relevant. After several weeks of this, some nurses stopped checking alerts at all, assuming they were probably false alarms. Then someone the system flagged amber attempted suicide. The nurse had seen the alert but dismissed it based on their previous experience that alerts were usually wrong.

What Went Right:

The implementation did catch some deteriorations early. One nurse, Elena (composite example), took alerts seriously despite frustration with false positives. She contacted Marcus, flagged as amber, who initially insisted he was fine. Elena gently explored further based on the alert prompting closer look. Marcus eventually disclosed increasing suicidal thoughts he'd been minimizing. Early intervention prevented crisis escalation.

The system identified patterns across populations that individual nurses wouldn't spot. It noticed that hospital discharge follow-ups were inconsistent and that patients discharged from inpatient care had significantly elevated crisis risk in weeks 2-4 post-discharge—a window where contact often lapsed. This population-level insight led to protocol changes improving transitions of care.

What They Changed:

Six months in, the team redesigned the implementation. They increased the threshold for alerts, accepting that they'd miss some true positives to reduce false positives to manageable levels. Instead of 180 alerts monthly, they received 40-50—still substantial but not overwhelming.

They created structured response protocols. Amber alerts triggered review of recent documentation and brief phone contact. Red alerts required face-to-face assessment within 24 hours. This prevented checkbox compliance and ensured meaningful clinical response.

They established a feedback loop. When nurses overrode algorithmic risk scores based on clinical judgment, they documented reasoning in detail. This data went back to system developers quarterly, allowing algorithm refinement based on what experienced nurses noticed that AI missed.

Lessons Learned:

1. Accuracy alone doesn't determine usefulness. A 75% accurate system generating unmanageable workload is less useful than a 60% accurate system with manageable alert volume.

2. Implementation matters as much as technology. The algorithm itself worked reasonably well. The failure was deploying it without adequate protocols for responding to alerts.

3. Staff trust is fragile. Once nurses concluded alerts were unreliable, rebuilding credibility took months of demonstrated improvement.

4. Clinical override must be supported, not discouraged. The best outcomes came when nurses used algorithmic flags as prompts for closer assessment but made final decisions based on clinical judgment.

5. Population insights can be as valuable as individual predictions. Even when the system incorrectly flagged specific patients, it identified system-level problems worth addressing.

7.2 Documentation AI Success

The Setting: A crisis resolution and home treatment team working 24/7 providing intensive home-based care. Typical shifts involved seeing 6-8 patients, each requiring comprehensive documentation. Nurses routinely stayed 60-90 minutes after shifts completing notes. Burnout was endemic.

What They Tried: Voice-to-text documentation software allowing nurses to dictate notes via smartphone immediately after appointments. The AI converted speech to formatted text, learning medical terminology and each nurse's documentation patterns over time. Notes required review and approval but eliminated typing.

Why It Worked:

The implementation was simple and addressed a clear pain point. Every nurse hated documentation. Anything reducing that burden would be welcomed if it actually worked and didn't create new problems.

Training was brief but effective. The trust brought in a specialist for half-day workshops teaching dictation techniques: speaking clearly, using structured formats, including punctuation commands. Nurses practiced with feedback until comfortable.

The technology itself was robust. Unlike earlier voice recognition requiring desktop computers, this worked on personal smartphones nurses already carried. Network connectivity was decent in most areas. The AI achieved over 95% accuracy after brief training on individual voices.

Most importantly, documentation time dropped dramatically. A study comparing time spent on notes before and after implementation showed nurses reduced documentation from average 25 minutes per patient to 8 minutes (Hammana et al., 2015). The 17-minute saving per patient meant staff left on time instead of staying late.

Unexpected Benefits:

Documentation quality improved in some ways. When typing, nurses often used templates with minimal personalization. When dictating, they naturally described what they observed rather than filling in forms. Notes became more narrative, capturing clinical nuance better.

Some nurses found dictation easier while driving between home visits. They could capture observations immediately after appointments rather than trying to remember details hours later. This improved accuracy and timeliness.

Team morale improved noticeably. Exit interviews with departing staff had consistently cited excessive documentation as a reason for leaving. After implementation, this complaint decreased significantly. The trust had better retention.

Problems That Emerged:

Privacy became a concern. Nurses dictating notes in cars or public spaces risked being overheard. The trust had to establish guidelines: dictate in private locations only, use headphones, don't include identifying information until reviewing notes privately.

Some nurses struggled with the format. They were used to writing and found speaking notes unnatural initially. A few never adapted and continued typing. The trust allowed both approaches rather than mandating voice recognition.

The AI occasionally misinterpreted critical words. "Denies suicidal ideation" became "endorses suicidal ideation" in one case due to poor audio quality. This wasn't caught during review, creating a dangerous documentation error. The trust implemented mandatory human review of risk-related statements to catch such errors.

Lessons Learned:

1. Target clear pain points. Documentation was universally hated. Solutions addressing widely-acknowledged problems get staff buy-in easily.

2. Make technology accessible. Smartphone-based solutions that don't require new hardware or complicated login procedures get adopted faster.

3. Provide adequate training upfront. The half-day workshop was essential. Without training, accuracy would have been poor and adoption would have failed.

4. Allow flexibility. Permitting nurses to continue typing if they preferred prevented resentment and acknowledged that different people work differently.

5. Monitor for new risks. Voice recognition created privacy concerns that hadn't existed with typed notes. Proactive guidance prevented problems.

6. Human review remains essential. The AI dramatically improved efficiency but introduced new error types. Quality control processes had to adapt.

7.3 Digital First Pathways

The Setting: An IAPT service implementing a digital-first pathway for mild-to-moderate depression and anxiety. The model directed new referrals to digital CBT (Wysa or SilverCloud) initially, with face-to-face therapy available for those who didn't improve or preferred human contact.

The Rationale: Waiting lists for face-to-face therapy were 16-20 weeks. Digital CBT could start immediately, providing something rather than nothing while people waited. Research suggested digital interventions were effective for mild-moderate presentations (Andrews et al., 2018). The service could potentially help more people with existing resources.

What Happened:

Uptake was good initially. About 70% of people offered digital CBT enrolled in the programs. This looked like success—far better than anticipated. The service congratulated itself on innovative care delivery.

But engagement rates told a different story. Only 35% of people who enrolled actually completed more than two sessions of digital content (Eysenbach, 2005). Most downloaded the app, looked at it once or twice, and never returned. Symptom improvement among completers was good, but the completion rate was dismal.

Dropout analysis revealed concerning patterns. People from deprived areas had significantly lower completion rates than affluent areas. Older adults dropped out more than younger people. Those with limited education struggled more than university graduates. The digital-first pathway was effectively providing excellent care to privileged populations while providing nothing to disadvantaged groups (Torous et al., 2020).

Patient feedback highlighted problems. Many people wanted human contact and felt fobbed off with an app. They'd gathered courage to seek help, and receiving automated content felt like rejection. Some explicitly said "I need a person, not a computer."

The service's outcome data looked good superficially—people who completed digital programs improved significantly. But this was survivorship bias. The only people included in outcome measurements were those who engaged. The 65% who dropped out disappeared from the data. The service was helping fewer people than before implementation despite higher enrollment numbers.

The Redesign:

One year in, the service changed the model substantially. Instead of purely digital-first, they offered choice: digital CBT with weekly brief phone support, traditional face-to-face therapy, or hybrid combining both. Most people chose hybrid or face-to-face.

They added human support to digital pathways. Patients using Wysa received brief weekly check-ins from therapists who reviewed their app activity, discussed progress, and provided accountability. Completion rates jumped to 62%—not perfect, but dramatically better (Erbe et al., 2017).

They identified and addressed digital exclusion. Patients without smartphones or data plans received tablets with pre-loaded content and WiFi access through community centers. Those with limited literacy received additional support understanding content.

They made face-to-face therapy available sooner for people who clearly weren't benefiting from digital approaches rather than insisting they complete digital programs first.

Lessons Learned:

1. Enrollment doesn't equal engagement. People signing up for digital programs doesn't mean they'll use them.

2. Digital-first can perpetuate inequity. If disadvantaged populations can't or won't engage with digital tools, you're creating two-tier care.

3. Patient preference matters enormously. Forcing digital approaches on people who want human contact generates resentment and disengagement.

4. Hybrid models work better than purely digital. Combining technology with human support produces higher engagement and better outcomes.

5. Measure what matters, not what's easy. Outcomes for completers is meaningless if most people don't complete. Include dropout rates in quality metrics.

6. Be willing to admit mistakes. The service initially defended the model despite evidence of problems. Acknowledging failure and redesigning was crucial to eventual success.

7.4 When AI Missed Crisis

The Scenario: A mental health trust implemented digital phenotyping for patients with bipolar disorder, monitoring smartphone data to detect early warning signs of mood episodes. The system tracked activity levels, sleep patterns, social contact, and phone use. Algorithms flagged concerning changes for clinical follow-up.

The Patient: Aisha, 29-year-old woman with bipolar I disorder, had been stable for 18 months on medication. She consented enthusiastically to digital monitoring, viewing it as a safety net. The system tracked her data continuously, establishing her baseline patterns.

What the Algorithm Saw:

Over four weeks, Aisha's data showed some changes but nothing dramatic. Sleep duration decreased slightly—from 7.5 hours average to 6.8 hours. Activity levels increased modestly. Social contact remained stable. Phone use increased somewhat, particularly evening hours. The algorithm calculated these changes at 32% probability of manic episode—amber category but not urgent.

Her CPN received a routine alert indicating minor risk elevation. Given caseload pressures, she planned to call Aisha at the next scheduled contact in 10 days. The algorithm hadn't flagged anything urgent enough to warrant immediate intervention.

What Actually Happened:

Aisha was entering a manic episode. The quantitative changes were modest, but qualitative changes were dramatic. She was sleeping less but felt more energetic. Increased phone use reflected grandiose business planning—she was messaging potential investors about a startup idea that was increasingly unrealistic. Increased activity reflected new gym routines and spontaneous travel plans she couldn't afford.

Her family noticed concerning changes. She was more talkative, making reckless decisions, and seemed irritable when questioned. They tried calling her CPN but reached voicemail. They didn't know the CPN had received an amber alert and was planning routine follow-up.

Eight days after the initial alert, Aisha presented to A&E in acute mania. She'd maxed out credit cards, quit her job, and started a relationship with someone she'd met online 24 hours earlier. Hospital admission was required. The manic episode that digital monitoring was supposed to catch early had progressed to full crisis.

What Went Wrong:

1. The algorithm measured quantity, not quality. Sleeping 45 minutes less sounds minor. But for Aisha, reduced sleep need was a cardinal symptom of mania. The algorithm couldn't distinguish between less sleep due to stress versus less sleep due to elevated mood.

2. The alert didn't convey urgency. Amber category among dozens of other alerts didn't prompt immediate action. The system lacked context showing this patient's pattern specifically.

3. Response protocols were inadequate. Amber alerts required action "within two weeks." For rapidly escalating mania, that's too slow.

4. Family weren't integrated. They noticed problems but had no clear pathway to communicate concerns. Digital monitoring created false confidence that systems were watching.

5. The algorithm couldn't measure what mattered most. Thought content, judgment, insight—the things that actually indicated mania—weren't captured by activity sensors.

What Changed:

The trust revised protocols substantially. Amber alerts for bipolar patients now triggered contact within 48 hours, recognizing that mood episodes can escalate rapidly. Red alerts required same-day assessment.

They established direct family contact routes. Relatives received information about how to report concerns urgently, separate from digital monitoring alerts. Clinical response integrated both algorithmic data and family observations.

They refined algorithms specifically for bipolar disorder, recognizing that different conditions need different thresholds. What counts as concerning change varies by diagnosis.

Most importantly, they reframed digital monitoring as one data source among many rather than comprehensive safety net. Clinical oversight increased rather than decreased with digital tools.

Lessons Learned:

1. Algorithms miss nuance. Quantitative data doesn't capture qualitative changes that are clinically significant.

2. Alert categorization must match clinical urgency. Generic green/amber/red systems may not fit specific conditions' needs.

3. Technology creates false confidence. Staff and families assumed monitoring meant Aisha was safe. It didn't.

4. Human oversight remains essential. Digital tools supplement clinical judgment; they don't replace it.

5. One-size-fits-all algorithms don't work. Different conditions need different approaches and thresholds.

6. Involve families actively. They often notice changes before algorithms do.

7.5 Top Ten Mistakes

Drawing from these cases and others, here are the most common implementation failures and how to avoid them:

1. Implementing technology without clear clinical rationale. Don't adopt AI because it's fashionable. Identify specific problems it might solve.

2. Ignoring workflow integration. Tools that require separate logins, duplicate data entry, or additional steps won't be used consistently.

3. Inadequate training. Expecting staff to figure out new systems independently guarantees poor adoption and misuse.

4. Treating AI outputs as definitive truth. Algorithms inform decisions; humans make them. Never abdicate clinical judgment to machines.

5. Overwhelming staff with alerts. High-sensitivity systems generating excessive false positives lead to alert fatigue and ignored warnings.

6. Measuring wrong outcomes. Track engagement, equity, actual clinical benefit—not just enrollment or completions among those who finish.

7. Assuming all patients can access digital tools. Digital exclusion is real and correlates with disadvantage. Provide alternatives.

8. Failing to involve frontline staff in planning. People implementing changes daily need input into how implementations work.

9. Implementing multiple changes simultaneously. Change one thing at a time. Otherwise you can't identify what works or what caused problems.

10. Giving up too quickly or persisting too long. Some implementations need time to work out issues. Others are fundamentally flawed and should be abandoned. Know the difference.

7.6 Moving Forward Informed

These case studies aren't meant to discourage AI adoption. They're meant to help you implement intelligently, anticipate problems, and learn from others' mistakes rather than repeating them.

Every implementation will face challenges. Technology will malfunction. Staff will resist. Algorithms will make errors. Patients will struggle with digital interfaces. That's normal. What matters is responding adaptively—recognizing problems, acknowledging them honestly, and making changes rather than defending failures.

The services that succeeded weren't those with perfect technology. They were those that listened to staff concerns, monitored outcomes honestly, involved patients in design, and adapted when approaches didn't work.

Your service's AI implementation will be imperfect. Make it as good as possible, monitor carefully, and improve continuously. That's how innovations become improvements rather than expensive mistakes.

Chapter 8.0: Data Hunger Explained

Every AI system in mental health care learned by consuming data—millions of patient records, clinical notes, treatment outcomes, demographic information, and behavioral patterns. These algorithms didn't emerge fully formed with clinical wisdom. They were trained on historical data, learning which patterns predicted which outcomes based on what happened to real patients in the past.

This creates a fundamental problem: **AI systems reflect the data they consumed, including all the biases, gaps, and inequalities embedded in that data** (Obermeyer et al., 2019). If training data overrepresents certain populations and underrepresents others, the algorithm works better for some patients than others. If historical data reflects discriminatory practices, the AI perpetuates discrimination. If documentation patterns vary by clinician bias, the algorithm learns those biases.

Understanding where AI systems get their data, how they learn from it, and what gets baked into their decision-making processes isn't optional knowledge for mental health nurses. It's essential for using these tools safely, recognizing their limitations, and advocating for patients when algorithms fail them.

8.1 Training Data Origins

AI algorithms learn from electronic health records, which means they're learning from documentation practices, coding decisions, and clinical judgments made by thousands of clinicians over years. This sounds comprehensive until you consider what's actually in those records (Char et al., 2018).

EHRs capture what clinicians documented, not necessarily what happened. If a patient experienced discrimination but the clinician didn't document it, that context is invisible to AI. If a symptom wasn't specifically asked about, it doesn't appear in structured data fields. If cultural factors influenced presentation but weren't noted, the algorithm has no way to account for them.

The data is also shaped by who had access to services. If mental health care has been less accessible to certain communities, those populations are underrepresented in training data. Algorithms trained primarily on white, middle-class patients don't perform as well for other groups—not because of something inherent to those groups, but because the AI hasn't seen enough examples to recognize their patterns (Gianfrancesco et al., 2018).

Research datasets used to develop AI tools often come from academic medical centers or well-resourced health systems. These settings serve specific populations—often more educated, more affluent, with better insurance coverage than the general population. An algorithm developed using data from a London teaching hospital may perform poorly when deployed in a community mental health service in Bradford serving a more diverse, economically disadvantaged population.

Consent for data use in research datasets is typically broad. Patients consented to their data being used for research but may not have understood it would train AI systems that make decisions about future patients. The consent forms signed a decade ago didn't mention machine learning because the technology didn't exist yet in healthcare. Now that data is being repurposed in ways patients never imagined (Vayena et al., 2015).

Here's a concrete example: A trust implements an AI risk assessment tool trained on data from 50,000 patients treated between 2010 and 2020. The training data includes demographic information, diagnoses, medications, appointment attendance, documented risk factors, and outcomes (hospitalizations, suicide attempts, disengagement from services).

The algorithm learns patterns like: patients who miss appointments and reduce medication adherence after relationship breakups show elevated crisis risk. That's useful. But it also learns patterns like: patients from certain postcodes have higher hospitalization rates. Is that because people in those areas have more severe illness, or because they have less community support, or because services in those areas have lower thresholds for admission, or because implicit bias influences admission decisions? The algorithm can't distinguish causation from correlation—it just learns that the pattern exists (Char et al., 2018).

Commercial data sources add another layer of complexity. Some AI companies supplement clinical data with information from social media, consumer purchases, web searches, or smartphone usage patterns. This data wasn't collected for healthcare purposes and wasn't subject to clinical governance or consent processes (Martinez-Martin et al., 2018).

A patient might have consented to their NHS records being used for AI development but never consented to their Facebook activity, Amazon purchases, or Google searches being incorporated. Yet some predictive models use exactly this kind of data, arguing it provides valuable behavioral insights not captured in clinical documentation.

The legal and ethical status of this practice remains contested. UK data protection law requires explicit consent for health data use. But the boundaries between "health data" and "lifestyle data" are fuzzy. Is your web search for "how to cope with depression" health data requiring medical-grade consent, or ordinary internet activity subject to standard terms of service? The answer matters enormously for what AI systems can legally access and learn from.

8.2 Data Bias Problems

Data bias occurs when training data doesn't represent the population the AI will serve, leading to systematically different performance across groups (Obermeyer et al., 2019). This isn't a minor technical issue—it's a major equity problem with real consequences for patients.

Consider a suicide risk algorithm trained primarily on data from younger adults. It learns patterns of suicide risk expression common in that age group—impulsive attempts, substance use, relationship crises, social media activity changes. Then it's deployed to assess risk in older adults, who show different patterns—more planned attempts, less substance involvement, medical illness as trigger, social isolation rather than social media changes. The algorithm misses risk in older adults because it never learned their patterns (Torous et al., 2020).

Gender bias appears in multiple ways. Historical data reflects the reality that women are diagnosed with depression more frequently than men, while men are diagnosed with substance use disorders more frequently. Are these true prevalence differences, or do diagnostic biases lead to over-diagnosing depression in women and under-diagnosing it in men? Algorithms trained on biased diagnostic data perpetuate those biases (Cirillo et al., 2020).

Men experiencing depression may present with irritability, anger, and risk-taking rather than sadness and tearfulness. If training data predominantly captured female depression presentations, the algorithm learned to recognize one pattern while missing another. The AI doesn't know it's biased—it's just learned what depression "looks like" based on who was diagnosed in the training data.

Racial and ethnic bias is perhaps the most documented and concerning form of algorithmic discrimination. A landmark 2019 study analyzing a commercial healthcare algorithm found it systematically underestimated illness severity in Black patients compared to white patients with the same objective health measures (Obermeyer et al., 2019).

The algorithm wasn't explicitly programmed to discriminate by race. The bias emerged because the AI used healthcare costs as a proxy for healthcare need—assuming patients who generated higher costs were sicker. But Black patients historically have less access to care, receive less treatment for the same conditions, and thus generate lower costs despite equal or greater illness severity. The algorithm interpreted lower costs as lower need, systematically deprioritizing Black patients for care programs.

In mental health, similar dynamics exist. Patients from minority ethnic communities face barriers accessing services, receive different treatments for the same presentations, and are more likely to enter care through crisis or criminal justice pathways rather than voluntary seeking of help (Halvorsrud et al., 2019). All of this creates training data patterns that don't reflect clinical need—they reflect systemic inequities in service access and delivery.

Socioeconomic bias appears when algorithms learn associations between poverty indicators and outcomes. Patients from deprived areas may have worse outcomes not because their mental illness is inherently more severe, but because they face more stressors (housing instability, food insecurity, unemployment), have less access to resources that support recovery, and experience more cumulative trauma. The algorithm sees the pattern—patients from certain postcodes do worse—but can't distinguish between illness severity and social determinants of health (Gianfrancesco et al., 2018).

An AI tool might flag patients from deprived areas as high-risk based purely on their postcode, not their clinical presentation. That could be helpful if it prompts intensive support for people facing socioeconomic adversity. Or it could be harmful if it creates self-fulfilling prophecies—people are expected to do poorly, so they receive less hopeful treatment, which contributes to poor outcomes.

Intersectionality multiplies these problems. A Black woman living in poverty faces compounded disadvantages that simple demographic categories don't capture. Algorithms typically treat demographic factors independently rather than understanding how multiple marginalized identities interact. The bias isn't additive—it's multiplicative (Buolamwini & Gebru, 2018).

8.3 Informed Consent Reimagined

Informed consent for algorithmic decision-making requires patients understand that AI influences their care, how it works, what data it uses, and what it means for their treatment (Vayena et al., 2015). That's far more complex than traditional consent for clinical procedures.

The conversation with Marcus, a 35-year-old man with anxiety (composite example), might go like this:

You: "I want to explain something about how we use technology in your care. Our system uses AI—artificial intelligence—to help assess which patients might be at risk of crisis. This means a computer program analyzes information from your records and gives us risk scores that help us prioritize who needs urgent attention."

Marcus: "What information does it use?"

You: "Everything in your NHS records—diagnoses, medications, appointment history, documented symptoms, previous hospitalizations if you've had any. It looks for patterns that historically meant someone was heading toward crisis. The algorithm was trained on data from thousands of patients who used our services before, learning which combinations of factors predicted problems."

Marcus: "Does it know I'm Black? Does that affect anything?"

You: "The system has access to demographic information including ethnicity. Ideally, this would help it recognize different presentations across populations. The concern is that algorithms sometimes perform differently for different groups depending on who was in the training data. We're supposed to monitor for bias, but it's something to be aware of."

Marcus: "Can I opt out?"

You: "The algorithmic risk scoring happens automatically as part of our electronic records system. You can't opt out of that while receiving care here. But you can ask questions about how it's used, see your risk scores if you want, and challenge decisions if you think the algorithm got it wrong. Your clinical care is ultimately based on my professional judgment, not what the computer says."

This conversation is honest about algorithmic involvement, explains data use clearly, acknowledges bias concerns, and clarifies limits on opting out. Many services don't have these conversations at all—patients receive AI-influenced care without knowing it exists (Wachter et al., 2017).

True informed consent would require explaining technical details most patients can't evaluate: which algorithm, trained on what data, achieving what accuracy, using which features. That's impossible without health data science literacy most people lack. So consent becomes more about transparency than genuine understanding—telling people AI is involved and giving them opportunities to ask questions, even if they can't fully grasp the technical implementation.

The right to explanation is partially protected under UK GDPR. Patients have the right to know when automated decision-making significantly affects them and to receive meaningful information about the logic involved (ICO, 2018). But "meaningful information" is legally vague, and mental health AI often involves clinical judgment combined with algorithmic input, making it unclear if the decision is sufficiently "automated" to trigger explanation rights.

A patient might challenge a decision to reduce their care frequency based partly on algorithmic low-risk scoring. Do they have the right to a detailed explanation of how the algorithm calculated that score? Current interpretation suggests they're entitled to know the algorithm was involved and the broad factors it considered, but not necessarily the precise mathematical weighting or model architecture, which may be proprietary.

8.4 Data Ownership Questions

Who owns patient data used to train AI systems? The legal answer is complicated. Patients own their personal data in the sense of having rights to access, correct, and request deletion under GDPR. But the NHS holds their health records as data controller, and researchers or AI developers may process that data as data processors with legitimate interests (ICO, 2018).

Once data is anonymized and aggregated for AI training, individual ownership becomes murky. You can't identify which specific patient's records contributed to an algorithm's behavior. The AI model itself—the mathematical relationships the algorithm learned—doesn't contain personal data in a form you could extract and attribute to individuals. But it was built from personal data, raising philosophical questions about ownership and benefit-sharing.

Commercial AI developers often train systems using NHS data, then sell the resulting products back to the NHS at substantial profit. Patients whose data trained the algorithm don't benefit financially. Some argue this is acceptable because AI development advances care for everyone. Others argue it's exploitative—privatizing gains from publicly-generated data without compensation or consent from data subjects (Powles & Hodson, 2017).

The Royal Free Hospital scandal illustrates these tensions. In 2015, the hospital provided 1.6 million patient records to DeepMind (Google) to develop an AI system for acute kidney injury detection. Patients weren't informed their data was being shared with a commercial tech company. The Information Commissioner ruled the data-sharing illegal because it lacked legal basis and appropriate consent (ICO, 2017).

This case established important precedents: commercial AI development using NHS data requires proper legal justification, patients should be informed about data-sharing arrangements, and "improving care" doesn't automatically justify all data uses. But implementation remains inconsistent across trusts.

Data sovereignty—the principle that individuals should control how their data is used—conflicts with AI development needs. Creating effective algorithms requires large datasets. If every patient must actively consent, participation rates may be too low to develop functional tools. But proceeding without explicit consent violates patient autonomy (Vayena et al., 2015).

Some propose a middle ground: patients are informed that NHS data may be used for AI development, have the right to opt out, but participation is default unless they actively refuse. This preserves autonomy while allowing research to proceed. Critics argue this exploits people's inertia and lack of technical knowledge—most patients don't understand AI well enough to make informed decisions about opting in or out.

Patient benefit should be central. If AI systems developed using patient data will eventually improve care for those same patients and their communities, there's a stronger ethical case than if the primary beneficiaries are shareholders of tech companies. NHS data-sharing agreements increasingly require that AI tools developed using NHS data must be made available to the NHS at reasonable cost rather than maximizing commercial profit.

8.5 Legal Responsibilities

GDPR (General Data Protection Regulation) governs all processing of personal data in the UK, including health data used for AI development (ICO, 2018). Key requirements for mental health nurses using AI tools:

Lawful basis for processing: AI systems processing patient data must have legal justification—typically either explicit consent, legal obligation, vital interests, public task, or legitimate interests. Mental health AI usually relies on "public task" (providing healthcare services) or "legitimate interests" (improving care quality). You need to understand which legal basis applies to the AI tools you use.

Special category data protections: Mental health information is "special category" data under GDPR, requiring additional safeguards. AI processing mental health data needs either explicit consent or must meet specific conditions like substantial public interest in health or social care. Most NHS AI implementations rely on public interest grounds, but this must be properly documented.

Data minimization: AI systems should only access data necessary for their purpose. If an algorithm assesses suicide risk, it shouldn't access irrelevant information about physical health conditions or family members' records unless clearly needed for the risk assessment. You should know what data your AI tools access and challenge unnecessary data collection.

Rights to access and rectification: Patients can request their data, including algorithmically-generated risk scores or recommendations. They can challenge inaccurate data. If a patient believes the algorithm is using incorrect information about them, you must facilitate correction of their records.

Right to restrict processing: In some circumstances, patients can request that AI systems stop processing their data. This might not be practically possible if the algorithm runs automatically on all records, but patients should know their rights and how to exercise them.

NHS data governance adds additional layers. Information governance training is mandatory for NHS staff. You're responsible for protecting patient confidentiality, using data only for legitimate care purposes, and reporting breaches. When AI tools are involved, these responsibilities extend to understanding what data the AI accesses and ensuring appropriate safeguards exist (NHS Digital, 2023).

Your personal legal responsibilities include:

Professional accountability: As a registered nurse, you remain accountable for all clinical decisions, even those influenced by AI recommendations. You can't blame the algorithm if something goes wrong—you're responsible for evaluating its output and deciding how to act (NMC, 2023).

Duty of candour: If AI-related errors contribute to harm, you must be open and honest with patients about what happened. This includes explaining the role of algorithmic recommendations in clinical decisions.

Data protection compliance: You must handle patient data in accordance with data protection law, including understanding how AI systems you use process that data and ensuring patients are informed about AI involvement in their care.

Record-keeping standards: You must document clearly when AI tools influence clinical decisions, noting what the algorithm recommended, your assessment, and your rationale for following or overriding algorithmic advice (NMC, 2023).

Breach reporting: If you become aware of data breaches involving AI systems—unauthorized access, data leaks, security failures—you must report them through appropriate channels promptly.

Elena, a community psychiatric nurse (composite example), discovered that a digital phenotyping app used by her patients was transmitting data to servers in a country without adequate data protection. This violated GDPR because personal data was being transferred outside the UK without appropriate safeguards. Elena reported this to her trust's data protection officer, who suspended use of the app pending security review.

Elena's action protected patients and demonstrated proper understanding of data protection responsibilities. Had she continued using the app after discovering the problem, she could have faced professional consequences for failing to safeguard patient data.

8.6 Essential Understanding

Data hunger drives AI development, but unexamined data consumption perpetuates biases, excludes marginalized populations, and creates systems that work better for some patients than others. Understanding where training data comes from, recognizing its limitations, and advocating for more representative data collection is part of your professional responsibility in an AI-augmented healthcare system.

The legal framework around data use for AI is evolving. GDPR provides baseline protections but wasn't written with machine learning in mind. NHS data governance policies are adapting to AI realities but implementation is inconsistent. Your role is ensuring patients' rights are protected, their data is used appropriately, and algorithmic systems serve rather than exploit the people they're meant to help.

The next chapter examines how data bias manifests in practice, what algorithmic discrimination looks like when it affects real patients, and what you can do about it.

Chapter 9.0: Algorithmic Bias Uncovered

An AI risk assessment tool works beautifully for white middle-class patients. It catches deteriorating mood in young professionals with reliable internet access, stable housing, and regular appointment attendance. But it systematically underestimates risk in homeless patients, asylum seekers, people from minority ethnic communities, and anyone whose life circumstances don't fit the patterns the algorithm learned from its predominantly white, stably-housed training data.

This isn't a hypothetical problem. It's happening right now in NHS trusts across the UK (Obermeyer et al., 2019). **Algorithmic bias**—systematic errors that produce unfair outcomes for certain groups—is one of the most serious ethical challenges in healthcare AI. And unlike individual clinician bias, which affects one patient at a time, algorithmic bias operates at scale, potentially disadvantaging thousands of patients simultaneously.

Your job as a mental health nurse includes recognizing when algorithms discriminate, advocating for patients harmed by biased systems, and pushing for equitable AI development. This chapter gives you the tools to do that effectively.

9.1 How AI Amplifies Disparity

Algorithmic bias doesn't emerge from malicious intent. Nobody programs AI to discriminate. Bias emerges because algorithms learn from historical data reflecting real-world inequalities, then perpetuate those inequalities in their predictions (Char et al., 2018).

Race-based disparities appear in multiple ways. A study analyzing healthcare algorithms in the United States found that Black patients were assigned lower risk scores than equally sick white patients, resulting in Black patients receiving less care despite equal need (Obermeyer et al., 2019). The algorithm used healthcare costs as a proxy for healthcare need, assuming patients who cost more required more care.

But this assumption ignored structural racism in healthcare access. Black patients historically receive less treatment for the same conditions due to discrimination, implicit bias, financial barriers, and mistrust of medical institutions based on historical exploitation. They generate lower healthcare costs not because they're less sick but because they receive less care. The algorithm interpreted lower costs as lower need, systematically under-prioritizing Black patients.

In UK mental health services, similar dynamics exist. Patients from Black Caribbean and Black African backgrounds have higher rates of compulsory admission under the Mental Health Act but lower rates of accessing talking therapies or community support (Halvorsrud et al., 2019). An algorithm trained on this data might "learn" that these populations need crisis intervention more than psychological therapy. Is that accurate clinical assessment, or is it learning patterns of institutional discrimination?

Gender bias manifests in diagnostic algorithms. Women are diagnosed with depression at roughly twice the rate of men (Albert, 2015). Is this true prevalence difference, or does it reflect diagnostic bias—doctors being quicker to diagnose depression in women while attributing similar symptoms in men to stress or normal reactions?

AI trained on biased diagnostic data perpetuates the bias. An algorithm assessing depression risk might be overly sensitive for women (generating false positives) and insufficiently sensitive for men (generating false negatives). Men experiencing depression but expressing it through anger, substance use, or risk-taking rather than sadness may be missed entirely because the algorithm learned depression "looks like" female presentations.

Socioeconomic bias appears when algorithms learn associations between poverty indicators and outcomes without understanding causation. Patients from deprived areas have worse mental health outcomes on average. But the reasons are complex—higher stress exposure, less access to protective factors, more cumulative trauma, poorer physical health, inadequate housing, food insecurity (Marmot et al., 2020).

An algorithm might flag patients from certain postcodes as high-risk based purely on address, essentially redlining mental health care. That could be helpful if it prioritizes intensive support for people facing socioeconomic adversity. Or it could create self-fulfilling prophecies—people are expected to do poorly, receive less hopeful treatment or reduced resources, and subsequently do worse.

Age bias works both directions. Algorithms may under-recognize mental health problems in older adults if training data predominantly included younger patients, missing the fact that depression in older people often presents differently—more somatic complaints, less acknowledgment of mood symptoms, more attribution to "normal aging." Conversely, algorithms might over-pathologize normal grief or adjustment reactions in older adults if training data conflated age with vulnerability.

Young people face different bias. Adolescent mental health presentations can be dismissed as "typical teenage angst" or developmental crisis rather than genuine illness. If algorithms are trained on data reflecting this dismissal, they perpetuate under-recognition of serious mental health problems in young people.

Intersectionality—the interaction of multiple marginalized identities—creates compounded disadvantage that algorithms handle poorly. A young Black woman from a deprived area faces race bias, gender bias, socioeconomic bias, and potentially age bias simultaneously. These don't add linearly—they multiply (Buolamwini & Gebru, 2018).

Algorithms typically treat demographic factors as independent variables, unable to capture how multiple oppressions interact. The error rate for facial recognition AI is 34% higher for darker-skinned women compared to lighter-skinned men, because most training data featured white males (Buolamwini & Gebru, 2018). Mental health AI likely shows similar intersectional accuracy gaps, though research documenting this is limited.

9.2 When Algorithms Fail

Let me describe what algorithmic discrimination looks like in practice through a composite case drawn from real implementations:

The Setting: An IAPT service implements an AI triage system to prioritize patients for initial assessment. The algorithm analyzes referral information and assigns urgency scores. High-urgency patients are assessed within one week. Moderate-urgency wait two to three weeks. Low-urgency wait up to eight weeks.

The Patient: Aisha, a 28-year-old Somali refugee who arrived in the UK three years ago. She's experiencing severe anxiety and depression related to trauma from her journey to the UK and ongoing asylum process. Her GP referral describes her symptoms clearly: panic attacks, nightmares, persistent low mood, suicidal thoughts without plan, significant functional impairment.

What the Algorithm Saw: The AI noted her symptoms but also processed other data points. No previous NHS mental health treatment history (she'd only been in the UK three years). Inconsistent GP attendance in her first two years (she didn't understand the appointment system initially and faced language barriers). Currently employed in low-wage precarious work. Living in temporary accommodation. Referral written by a GP who doesn't speak her first language, potentially missing nuance in her presentation.

The algorithm compared Aisha's profile to its training data showing which referrals resulted in appointment attendance, treatment engagement, and symptom improvement. Patients with her profile—refugee/asylum seeker background, housing instability, employment precarity, short UK residency—had lower completion rates in historical data. The algorithm interpreted these factors as predicting low engagement likelihood, assigned her moderate urgency, and recommended a three-week wait.

What Actually Happened: Aisha waited three weeks for assessment. During that time, her housing situation deteriorated (her landlord gave notice). Her symptoms worsened significantly. She presented to A&E in crisis, was briefly hospitalized, and eventually received intensive support that should have been provided initially.

The Post-Implementation Review: The service analyzed triage patterns and discovered shocking disparities. Patients with refugee or asylum seeker backgrounds were systematically assigned lower urgency scores than UK-born patients with identical symptom presentations. The algorithm had learned from historical data showing lower treatment completion rates in this population—but hadn't been programmed to understand *why* those rates were lower.

The lower completion wasn't due to less severe illness or less motivation for treatment. It reflected systemic barriers: language difficulties accessing services designed for English speakers, immigration-related crises disrupting appointment attendance, housing instability making consistent engagement difficult, cultural differences in help-seeking and symptom expression that services hadn't adequately accommodated (Satinsky et al., 2019).

The algorithm interpreted these barriers as patient characteristics predicting poor outcomes, then deprioritized this population for timely care—thereby ensuring continued poor outcomes. The AI wasn't recognizing that historical patterns reflected service failures, not patient deficits.

9.3 Identifying Bias

Red flags indicating your AI tools may be biased:

Disparate impact: Certain demographic groups consistently receive different risk scores, triage priorities, or treatment recommendations despite similar clinical presentations. Check if patients from minority ethnic backgrounds, deprived areas, or other marginalized groups are systematically over- or under-identified by algorithms (Gianfrancesco et al., 2018).

Pattern mismatch: Algorithm recommendations don't match your clinical assessment for specific populations. If you notice the AI consistently under-rates risk for older adults or over-rates crisis probability for young Black men, that's evidence of potential bias requiring investigation.

Worse outcomes in subgroups: Track outcomes by demographics. If patients from certain groups have worse outcomes despite similar algorithmic risk scores, the algorithm may be miscalibrated for them. For example, if patients flagged as "low risk" from one ethnic group are hospitalized at higher rates than "low risk" patients from another group, the algorithm isn't working equally well for both.

Data representation gaps: Ask developers what data trained the algorithm. If training data vastly underrepresents populations your service treats, expect poor performance for those groups. An algorithm trained on 90% white patients will perform worse for minority ethnic patients (Rajkomar et al., 2018).

Lack of validation across subgroups: Responsible AI development includes testing algorithm performance separately for different demographic groups. If developers can't show you accuracy metrics broken down by race, gender, age, and socioeconomic status, they haven't adequately evaluated bias (Char et al., 2018).

Opaque decision-making: "Black box" algorithms that can't explain their reasoning make bias detection nearly impossible. If you can't see which factors influenced a risk score, you can't identify when the algorithm weights factors inappropriately (Rudin, 2019).

Feedback loops: Biased algorithms can create self-fulfilling prophecies. If an AI systematically under-prioritizes care for a population, they receive less service, have worse outcomes, which "validates" the algorithm's prediction that they don't benefit from intervention, reinforcing future under-prioritization. This feedback loop amplifies initial bias over time (Obermeyer et al., 2019).

Practical steps for bias detection:

Conduct disparity audits: Regularly analyze algorithmic outputs by demographic groups. Calculate what percentage of each group receives high-risk flags, urgent triage priority, or treatment recommendations. Compare this to objective need measures. If 10% of white patients are flagged high-risk but 25% of Black patients are, investigate why.

Track clinical overrides: When nurses override algorithmic recommendations based on clinical judgment, document patterns. If you consistently override low-risk scores for specific populations because the algorithm missed important factors, that's evidence of systematic bias.

Listen to patients: Ask patients from marginalized groups about their experiences with AI-influenced care. Do they feel fairly assessed? Have they encountered situations where algorithms seemed to misunderstand their presentations? Patient-reported experiences can reveal bias that metrics miss (Laranjo et al., 2020).

Involve diverse stakeholders: Include people from affected communities in AI evaluation. They'll recognize cultural blind spots or biased assumptions that developers and clinicians might miss.

9.4 Advocacy Strategies

What nurses can do about algorithmic bias:

Document and report: When you encounter apparent bias, document specific cases clearly: patient demographics, algorithmic recommendation, your clinical assessment, outcome. Report through clinical governance channels, not just informally. Create a record that can drive system-level change (Char et al., 2018).

Challenge procurement decisions: When your trust considers purchasing AI tools, advocate for bias testing as a procurement requirement. Demand that vendors provide:

- Demographic breakdown of training data
- Accuracy metrics by subgroup
- Third-party bias audit results
- Plans for ongoing monitoring and mitigation

Advocate for transparent algorithms: Push for interpretable AI systems that explain their reasoning rather than black-box tools that hide decision-making processes. You can't identify or challenge bias you can't see (Rudin, 2019).

Participate in governance: Join AI oversight committees, digital health working groups, or equality and diversity committees evaluating AI implementations. Ensure frontline clinical voices shape policy.

Educate colleagues: Many healthcare professionals don't understand algorithmic bias or know how to recognize it. Share knowledge, raise awareness, and build collective capacity for critical evaluation of AI tools.

Connect with patient advocacy groups: Organizations representing marginalized communities have strong interest in equitable AI. Partner with them to amplify concerns and push for change.

Demand disaggregated data: Insist that your service tracks AI system performance by demographic groups, not just overall. Without disaggregated data, disparities remain invisible.

Support diverse AI development teams: Homogeneous development teams create algorithms reflecting their own blind spots. Advocate for diverse hiring in AI development, including people with lived experience of mental illness and marginalization (West et al., 2019).

Use your professional voice: Write to the Royal College of Nursing, RCNi forums, or nursing journals about algorithmic bias experiences. Professional organizations can pressure vendors and trusts in ways individual nurses cannot.

James, a senior CPN (composite example), noticed that an AI scheduling tool consistently allocated shorter appointment times to patients with interpreters, apparently "learning" from historical data that interpreted appointments overran so needed extra buffer time. But the algorithm created 15-minute appointment slots for interpreted sessions versus 30 minutes for English-speaking patients.

James documented this pattern, calculated that it meant patients with interpreters received half the contact time, and presented findings to the trust's AI steering committee. His evidence—showing clear disadvantage to patients with language barriers—led to algorithm modification ensuring equal appointment duration regardless of language.

That's effective advocacy: identifying specific bias, documenting impact, presenting evidence through appropriate channels, and achieving concrete change.

9.5 Cultural Competence Limits

Can AI be culturally competent? That's a profound question with no simple answer.

Cultural competence in human care requires understanding how cultural background influences symptom expression, help-seeking, therapeutic expectations, and recovery pathways (Kirmayer et al.,

2018). It requires adapting communication, recognizing cultural strengths, and avoiding imposing dominant-culture assumptions.

AI lacks cultural understanding in any meaningful sense. Algorithms can be programmed to account for cultural differences if developers know what those differences are and have data representing them. But AI can't develop cultural sensitivity through experience, can't ask culturally-informed questions, can't recognize when cultural context changes the meaning of behaviors.

Some attempts at "culturally-sensitive AI" have made things worse. One symptom checker included culturally-specific symptom descriptions for different ethnic groups but based these on stereotypes rather than evidence, reinforcing problematic assumptions (Chen et al., 2021).

The representation problem is fundamental. AI trained predominantly on Western, white populations learns Western, white patterns as "normal." Everything else becomes deviation or error. Creating truly culturally competent AI would require:

- Massive training datasets from diverse populations
- Cultural expertise in algorithm design
- Ongoing testing across cultural groups
- Mechanisms for incorporating cultural knowledge that can't be captured in quantifiable data

None of that exists at scale (West et al., 2019).

Linguistic issues compound problems. Most mental health AI operates in English. Even when translated, cultural concepts don't translate cleanly. The word "depression" doesn't have equivalent meaning across cultures. Some languages lack direct translations for anxiety, trauma, or mental illness concepts central to Western psychiatry.

NLP algorithms analyzing text or speech in non-English languages perform poorly because most training data is English. Accent recognition systems struggle with non-native speakers. Voice analysis AI detecting depression from speech patterns was trained on American English speakers and performs worse on other accents and languages (Cummins et al., 2015).

Realistic goals for equitable AI aren't full cultural competence—that's probably unachievable with current technology. But we can demand:

- Training data including diverse populations
- Testing that documents performance differences across groups
- Honest limitations stated clearly
- Human oversight that brings cultural competence algorithms lack
- Ongoing monitoring and refinement to reduce disparities

Perfect equity may be impossible, but we can refuse to accept AI systems that actively increase inequalities.

9.6 Moving Toward Equity

Algorithmic bias isn't inevitable. It results from choices—about what data to collect, which populations to include, how to define outcomes, whether to test for disparities, and whether to act on evidence of bias. Different choices produce different, more equitable outcomes (Rajkomar et al., 2018).

Your role isn't building algorithms—that's for data scientists. Your role is demanding that algorithms serve all patients fairly, recognizing when they don't, advocating for those harmed by biased systems, and refusing to accept inequity as the price of innovation.

Mental health nursing has a long history of advocating for marginalized patients against systems that disadvantage them. Algorithmic bias is the latest iteration of that old challenge. Your professional values—dignity, respect, equity, advocacy—apply just as much to AI systems as to any other aspect of care.

Chapter 10.0: Privacy and Patient Trust

A mental health chatbot gets hacked. Thousands of patient conversations—people discussing suicidal thoughts, trauma histories, relationship problems, medication side effects—are dumped on the dark web. Names, email addresses, sometimes phone numbers are included. Patients discover their most vulnerable moments have become public data.

This isn't hypothetical scaremongering. It happened. Multiple times. Mental health apps have experienced data breaches exposing intimate patient information to unauthorized access (Huckvale et al., 2019). And these were apps that claimed to prioritize security, that assured users their data was protected, that promised confidentiality comparable to traditional therapy.

Privacy and security in AI-augmented mental health care are fundamentally different from traditional clinical confidentiality. Your paper notes locked in a filing cabinet can't be hacked from another continent. Your verbal conversation with a patient doesn't create a permanent digital record accessible to anyone with the right technical skills. AI systems process and store data in ways that create new vulnerabilities—and many patients don't understand the risks they're accepting (Martinez-Martin et al., 2020).

Your role includes explaining these risks honestly, helping patients make informed decisions about digital mental health tools, and maintaining trust even as technology creates new threats to confidentiality.

10.1 When Security Fails

Data breaches in mental health apps happen with alarming frequency. A 2019 analysis of mental health apps found that 29 out of 36 transmitted data to third parties without adequately informing users, many had no privacy policy at all, and security practices were often woefully inadequate (Huckvale et al., 2019).

The consequences are severe. Mental health information is particularly sensitive—stigmatized, potentially damaging if disclosed, and precisely the kind of data people need to trust will remain confidential. A breach exposing mental health records creates risks beyond typical medical data breaches: employment discrimination, relationship damage, social stigma, and psychological harm from violation of trust (Torous & Roberts, 2017).

What happens in practice: Wysa, a mental health chatbot used by millions including NHS patients, experienced a security vulnerability in 2019 that could have exposed user conversations. The company fixed the issue before major exploitation occurred, but the incident highlighted how digital therapeutic tools create permanent records of intimate conversations that traditional therapy wouldn't (Huckvale et al., 2019).

Talkspace, another therapy app, faced criticism for data practices including sharing de-identified user information with third parties for advertising purposes. "De-identified" data isn't actually anonymous—research shows that combining a few data points (age, gender, location, diagnosis) can often re-identify specific individuals (Rocher et al., 2019). Someone's "anonymous" therapy transcripts can become identifiable with modest effort.

The weakest link in mental health AI security is often not the core algorithm but the surrounding infrastructure: how data is transmitted, where it's stored, who has access, how long it's retained, and what happens during disposal. Many AI tools upload patient data to cloud servers for processing. Those servers may be located in countries with weaker data protection laws than the UK. The data transmission may not be adequately encrypted. Server security may be compromised (Huckvale et al., 2019).

Insider threats are another vulnerability. Healthcare workers with access to AI systems can potentially access far more patient information than traditional paper systems allowed. An EHR might let you view records for thousands of patients if security controls are inadequate. Digital phenotyping data could reveal intimate details about people's lives—where they go, who they contact, when they sleep. The potential for misuse is substantial (Sujan et al., 2019).

Elena, a community psychiatric nurse (composite example), discovered a colleague had been accessing patient records without clinical justification, looking up information about acquaintances whose mental health status she was curious about. The electronic system logged the inappropriate access, leading to investigation and dismissal. But the breach had already occurred—confidential information had been viewed without authorization.

Chatbot-specific vulnerabilities include the permanence of conversations. When you speak with a patient face-to-face, there's no recording unless you explicitly create one. When someone uses a therapeutic chatbot, every word they type is captured, stored, and potentially analyzable. Most users don't fully grasp this permanence or consider who might access those records in the future (Laranjo et al., 2018).

10.2 The Trust Conversation

Explaining AI and data use to patients requires balancing transparency with comprehensibility. Technical details about encryption protocols and server architecture mean nothing to most people. But patients need enough information to make informed decisions about whether to engage with AI tools.

Here's how that conversation might go with Marcus, a 42-year-old man considering using a digital therapeutic app (composite example):

You: "Before you start using this app, I want to explain what happens to your data—the information you'll share through the app. Everything you type gets stored on secure servers. The company says the data is encrypted, which means it's scrambled so unauthorized people can't read it. But the company itself can access your conversations for quality improvement and to train their AI to work better."

Marcus: "So they're reading what I write?"

You: "Not necessarily reading every conversation personally, but their staff can access them. The app's privacy policy says they use de-identified data—meaning they remove your name and identifying details—to improve their algorithms. But 'de-identified' doesn't always mean truly anonymous. Sometimes it's possible to figure out who someone is even without their name, by combining other details."

Marcus: "Can other people see my information?"

You: "The company says they don't sell personal data to advertisers. But they might share anonymized information with research partners or use it internally in ways you might not expect. The privacy policy is long and complicated—most people don't read it fully. The reality is that when you use digital tools, you're trading some privacy for convenience and access."

Marcus: "What if there's a data breach? What if hackers get in?"

You: "That's a real risk. No system is completely secure. Mental health apps have been hacked before. If that happened, your conversations could potentially become public. The company would be legally required to notify you if there's a breach, but by then the damage is done. That's why I'm being honest about the risks before you decide whether to use this."

Marcus: "Is it safer than talking to you?"

You: "Our conversations are documented in NHS records, which have strong security protections under UK law. The NHS has had data breaches too—no system is perfect—but the legal framework and security standards are generally stronger than most app companies. The trade-off is that the app is available 24/7 when I'm not, which might be valuable for you. You need to decide if that convenience is worth the additional privacy risks."

This conversation is honest about vulnerabilities, doesn't oversell security, acknowledges uncertainty, and respects Marcus's right to make informed decisions. Many services don't have these conversations at all—patients are given app recommendations without understanding what they're consenting to (Torous & Roberts, 2017).

Conversation starters for different scenarios:

Introducing digital phenotyping: "This monitoring app tracks data from your phone—things like how much you're moving, your sleep patterns, and general phone use. It doesn't read your messages or see who you're contacting, but it does collect information about your behavioral patterns. That data gets analyzed by an algorithm looking for concerning changes. The benefit is early detection if you're deteriorating. The trade-off is constant monitoring, which some people find intrusive or anxiety-provoking."

Explaining algorithmic risk assessment: "Our system uses AI to assess which patients might be at elevated risk of crisis. It analyzes information from your records—diagnoses, medications, appointment patterns, documented symptoms. The algorithm looks for combinations of factors that historically meant someone was heading toward problems. This helps us prioritize who needs urgent attention. But algorithms can be wrong, and they sometimes work better for some groups than others. My clinical judgment always takes priority over what the computer says."

Discussing data sharing: "Your NHS records might be used—in anonymized form—to train AI systems that could help future patients. You have the right to opt out of this kind of data sharing for research and AI development. If you want to opt out, I can help you with that process. The trade-off is that opting out might slow the development of tools that could eventually benefit you or people like you."

10.3 Building Trust

Trust in AI-augmented care requires demonstrating that technology serves patients' interests rather than just institutional efficiency or corporate profit (Laranjo et al., 2018). Vulnerable populations—people with severe mental illness, trauma survivors, those who've experienced discrimination—are particularly cautious about systems that feel surveillance-oriented.

Transparency is foundational. Patients should know when AI is involved in their care, how it influences decisions, what data it uses, and how to challenge algorithmic recommendations. Hidden AI creates mistrust when patients discover it later (Wachter et al., 2017).

James, a 38-year-old man with PTSD (composite example), discovered after three months of treatment that an AI system had been analyzing his appointment attendance and medication collection patterns to predict disengagement risk. He was furious that nobody had told him. He felt surveilled, manipulated, and betrayed—his trust in the service severely damaged. The trust could have been preserved with a simple conversation explaining the system upfront.

Control matters enormously. When patients feel AI is something done *to* them without their input, it feels oppressive. When they feel it's a tool they can choose to use or not, it feels empowering. Offering choices—even limited ones—builds trust (Torous et al., 2020).

Offer options like: "Some people find digital tools helpful between our sessions. Others prefer not to mix technology with therapy.

What feels right for you?" This respects autonomy rather than imposing solutions.

Demonstrated benefit builds trust over time. If digital tools genuinely help patients feel better, they'll trust them more. If tools are frustrating, don't work as promised, or feel like they're serving institutional needs rather than patient needs, trust erodes (Musiat et al., 2014).

Track whether patients find AI tools helpful. Ask explicitly: "Has the app been useful? Is it worth the time you're putting into it? If not, let's try something different." This shows you care about their experience, not just their compliance.

Cultural sensitivity in AI implementation acknowledges that different communities have different relationships with technology, surveillance, and institutional trust. Communities with histories of medical exploitation or discrimination may be particularly wary of AI systems (Benjamin, 2019).

For asylum seekers, refugees, or people with immigration concerns, digital monitoring can feel dangerously similar to surveillance by immigration enforcement. For Black communities in the UK, algorithmic bias in policing creates warranted skepticism about all algorithmic systems. For older adults or people from working-class backgrounds, technology itself may feel alienating or inaccessible.

Acknowledge these realities: "I know some people worry about data and privacy, especially if they've had bad experiences with systems that didn't protect them. If you have concerns, I want to hear them. We can work within your comfort level."

Safeguarding vulnerable patients requires extra caution. People experiencing psychosis, severe depression, or active suicidal ideation may not be able to make fully informed decisions about digital tools. In these situations, prioritize protecting patients over implementing technology (Torous & Roberts, 2017).

Someone in acute crisis doesn't need a chatbot—they need immediate human support. Offering digital therapeutics to severely unwell patients can feel like abandonment dressed up as innovation. Be clear about when technology is appropriate and when it isn't.

10.4 When Patients Refuse

The backlash risk is real. Some patients hate AI involvement in their care. They find it dehumanizing, intrusive, creepy, or fundamentally incompatible with what they need from mental health support (Laranjo et al., 2018). Forcing AI on reluctant patients damages therapeutic relationships and may drive people away from services entirely.

Common objections:

"I don't want a computer involved in my mental health." This is about preferring human connection over technological mediation. It's a valid preference, not resistance to be overcome. Respect it. Ensure face-to-face care remains available for people who prefer it.

"I don't trust where my data goes." Given documented data breaches and privacy violations, this is rational skepticism, not paranoia. Don't dismiss it. Acknowledge the reality of data risks and offer as much control as possible over what data is collected and how it's used.

"The AI doesn't understand me." Algorithms struggle with complexity, nuance, and lived experience that doesn't fit neat categories. Patients from marginalized backgrounds often feel—correctly—that AI systems weren't designed for them. Validate this concern and ensure human clinicians remain central to care (Benjamin, 2019).

"It feels like you're trying to replace real care with cheap technology." If services are using AI primarily to manage demand rather than improve quality, patients notice. Be honest about why AI is being implemented. If it's a cost-saving measure, don't pretend it's primarily for patient benefit.

"I've heard AI is biased." As we discussed in Chapter 9.0, algorithmic bias is real and well-documented. Don't gaslight patients by dismissing these concerns. Acknowledge bias exists, explain what your service does to monitor for it, and commit to prioritizing clinical judgment over algorithmic recommendations when they conflict.

How to respond when patients refuse AI involvement:

Normalize the refusal: "That's completely understandable. AI in healthcare is new and raises legitimate concerns. You're not required to use digital tools if they don't feel right for you."

Offer alternatives: "Let's focus on what does work for you. We have face-to-face options, phone support, and traditional written materials if those feel more comfortable."

Don't penalize: Never make patients feel they're receiving inferior care because they refused AI tools. If services deprioritize patients who won't engage with technology, that's coercive and unethical.

Stay open: "If you change your mind later, the option is there. If you never change your mind, that's fine too."

Document appropriately: Note in records that AI tools were offered and declined, and the rationale. This protects both you and the patient. Don't frame refusal as "non-compliance" or "resistance to treatment"—frame it as patient preference.

10.5 Balancing Innovation and Safety

Innovation in mental health care is genuinely needed. Services are overwhelmed, access is inadequate, and traditional models can't meet population need with available resources. AI offers potential solutions to real problems (Torous et al., 2020).

But innovation can't come at the cost of patient safety, privacy, autonomy, or trust. The rush to implement AI sometimes prioritizes institutional needs over patient rights. Your job is maintaining that balance—supporting beneficial innovation while protecting patients from harm.

Safeguarding principles for AI implementation:

Patient benefit first: Only implement AI tools that genuinely serve patient interests, not just organizational efficiency or cost reduction.

Informed consent: Ensure patients understand AI involvement in their care and have meaningful opportunities to refuse without penalty.

Human oversight: Never allow algorithms to make clinical decisions autonomously. AI informs; humans decide.

Equity monitoring: Track whether AI systems work equally well across all patient populations. Address disparities proactively.

Privacy protection: Demand robust data security, minimal data collection, and clear limits on data use and sharing.

Transparency: Make AI involvement visible rather than hidden. Explain how systems work in language patients can understand.

Reversibility: Maintain non-digital alternatives so patients can opt out of AI-mediated care without losing access to services.

Continuous evaluation: Monitor outcomes, side effects, and patient experiences. Be willing to discontinue AI tools that don't deliver promised benefits or create unacceptable harms.

The goal isn't rejecting innovation—it's ensuring innovation serves rather than exploits patients. Technology that erodes trust, violates privacy, or increases inequity isn't innovative healthcare—it's corporate profiteering dressed up in the language of progress.

10.6 Core Principles

Privacy and security in AI-augmented mental health care are active challenges requiring ongoing attention, not problems solved once and forgotten. Data breaches will continue happening. New vulnerabilities will emerge. Patient trust will be tested repeatedly.

Your responsibility is staying informed about risks, being honest with patients about what they're consenting to, advocating for robust privacy protections, and maintaining the therapeutic relationship as the foundation of care—with or without technological augmentation.

Trust is hard to build and easy to destroy. Every honest conversation about AI limitations, every instance of respecting patient autonomy, every time you prioritize patient interests over institutional convenience—these build trust that makes AI-augmented care possible. Lose that trust, and even beneficial technology becomes impossible to implement ethically.

Chapter 11.0: The Accountability Question

An AI risk calculator flags a patient as low-risk. You agree with the assessment and schedule routine follow-up. Three days later, the patient attempts suicide. Who's responsible? You, for accepting the algorithmic recommendation? The algorithm developers, for creating a tool that missed the warning signs? Your trust, for implementing an inadequately tested system? The patient, for not disclosing suicidal intent?

Accountability in AI-augmented healthcare is legally and ethically complex. Traditional models of medical negligence assume human clinicians make decisions and bear responsibility for outcomes. AI disrupts this by inserting algorithmic recommendations into clinical decision-making, creating ambiguity about where responsibility lies when things go wrong (Price, 2017).

You need to understand the legal framework, your professional obligations, how to document AI-influenced decisions defensibly, and what protection your indemnity insurance actually provides. This isn't abstract theory—these questions will determine your legal exposure if AI systems you use contribute to patient harm.

11.1 Legal Liability Landscape

Who's legally responsible when AI gets clinical decisions wrong depends on multiple factors: the nature of the error, the role AI played in decision-making, whether there was human oversight, and how adequately the system was tested and implemented (Price, 2017).

Three potential parties bear liability:

You—the clinician: Under UK law, registered nurses remain professionally accountable for all clinical decisions, including those influenced by AI recommendations (NMC, 2023). You can't blame the algorithm if you followed its recommendation and it proved wrong. Your duty is exercising independent clinical judgment, which includes critically evaluating AI outputs rather than accepting them uncritically.

If you override algorithmic recommendations based on sound clinical reasoning, you're generally protected even if the outcome is poor—you exercised judgment, considered available information, and made a defensible decision. If you blindly follow AI recommendations despite clinical red flags suggesting the algorithm is wrong, you're likely liable for negligent failure to exercise professional judgment (Mulholland & Ulahannan, 2020).

The AI developer/vendor: Companies that create and sell AI tools can potentially be held liable for faulty products causing harm. But proving liability is difficult. You'd need to show the algorithm failed to perform as advertised, contained design flaws, or wasn't adequately tested. Most AI vendors disclaim liability through terms of service stating their tools support rather than replace clinical judgment (Price, 2017).

Regulatory pathways matter here. AI tools classified as medical devices under MHRA regulations carry higher accountability standards than unregulated wellness apps. Developers of medical device AI have clearer legal obligations regarding safety, effectiveness, and post-market surveillance (MHRA, 2023).

The healthcare organization: Trusts bear vicarious liability for staff actions and responsibility for system-level failures. If a trust implements inadequately tested AI, provides insufficient training, or creates workflows where staff can't effectively oversee algorithms, the organization shares liability for resulting harm (Mulholland & Ulahannan, 2020).

Emerging case law on AI in healthcare is limited but growing. Most cases settle out of court, preventing legal precedents from developing. But patterns are emerging:

When harm results from AI use, legal analysis focuses on whether human clinicians had adequate opportunity to detect and correct algorithmic errors. Courts generally hold that humans retain ultimate responsibility for clinical decisions, meaning you can't avoid liability by claiming you were "just following the algorithm" (Price, 2017).

A hypothetical case illustrates the principles: Elena, a CPN, uses an AI risk assessment tool that flags Diego, a 45-year-old patient, as low-risk. Elena spends 15 minutes with Diego, conducts a brief assessment, and schedules him for routine follow-up in four weeks based largely on the algorithmic low-risk score. Diego mentions feeling hopeless and having passive suicidal thoughts but no plan. Elena documents this but doesn't escalate care because the AI score was reassuring.

Diego attempts suicide two weeks later. In subsequent investigation, Elena's documentation shows she noted warning signs but deferred to the algorithmic assessment over her clinical observations. She's found to have failed in her professional duty to exercise independent judgment. The algorithm may have been flawed, but Elena's responsibility was critically evaluating its output—which she didn't adequately do (Mulholland & Ulahannan, 2020).

Contrast this with James, another CPN, using the same AI tool. It flags Marcus as low-risk, but James's clinical assessment reveals recent relationship breakdown, increasing alcohol use, and hopelessness. James documents clearly: "Algorithm scores low-risk based on historical factors, but current presentation shows concerning changes. Overriding algorithmic assessment. Escalating to urgent care." Marcus receives immediate support.

If Marcus still deteriorates, James has documented sound clinical reasoning for his decisions. He considered the AI input but exercised independent judgment when clinical presentation didn't match algorithmic prediction. That's defensible practice (NMC, 2023).

11.2 Clinical Negligence Framework

Clinical negligence in AI contexts follows the Bolam test: would a responsible body of medical professionals have acted similarly in the circumstances? The question becomes: would a reasonable mental health nurse have accepted the algorithmic recommendation, or would they have recognized it was wrong and overridden it? (Mulholland & Ulahannan, 2020).

Elements of negligence:

Duty of care: You owe patients a duty to provide care meeting professional standards. This applies whether you're using AI tools or not.

Breach of duty: You breached that duty if you failed to meet the standard expected of a reasonably competent practitioner. Using AI doesn't lower the standard of care—you're still expected to exercise appropriate clinical judgment (Price, 2017).

Causation: The breach must have caused harm. If you negligently accepted an incorrect algorithmic assessment, and that directly led to inadequate care causing patient harm, causation is established.

Harm: Actual damage must have occurred. Near-misses where harm was avoided don't constitute negligence in legal terms, though they may trigger professional conduct reviews.

AI-specific defenses:

"I was following trust protocol" may provide some protection if protocols specifically instructed you to defer to algorithmic recommendations. But protocols mandating uncritical acceptance of AI outputs are themselves negligent—they violate the professional requirement for nurses to exercise independent judgment (NMC, 2023).

"The algorithm was certified/approved" doesn't eliminate your responsibility. Even MHRA-approved medical devices require appropriate use and clinical oversight. Approval means the device meets safety standards—not that it's infallible or appropriate for every situation.

"I wasn't trained adequately" might shift liability toward your employer but doesn't fully absolve you. Nurses have professional responsibility to seek training and not practice beyond competence. If you felt inadequately trained to use AI tools safely, you should have raised concerns and sought training before using them clinically.

Documentation standards when using AI are crucial for defending your practice:

Record what the algorithm recommended: Note the specific risk score, triage priority, or clinical recommendation the AI generated. "System flagged patient as amber-risk with 58% crisis probability."

Record your independent assessment: Document your clinical findings separately from AI outputs. "Mental state examination shows low mood, poor sleep, anhedonia. Patient reports passive suicidal ideation without plan. Appears tired but engaged well in conversation."

Record your decision-making: Explain how you integrated algorithmic recommendations with your clinical judgment. "Algorithm assessment consistent with my clinical impression. Scheduling routine follow-up in two weeks with plan for earlier contact if symptoms worsen."

Or: "Algorithm scores low-risk, but clinical presentation shows concerning changes not captured in structured data. Overriding algorithmic assessment and escalating care."

Record rationale for any clinical override: When you disagree with AI recommendations, document why clearly. "Algorithm prioritizes this patient as low-urgency based on lack of recent service contact. However, GP referral describes acute deterioration following bereavement. Clinical urgency doesn't match algorithmic assessment. Scheduling urgent assessment within 48 hours."

This documentation demonstrates you exercised independent judgment, considered multiple information sources, and made reasoned decisions. That's defensible practice even if outcomes are poor (NMC, 2023).

11.3 Professional Indemnity Coverage

Your professional indemnity insurance—whether through your union, RCN membership, or independent provider—needs to cover AI-related claims. Many nurses don't realize that standard indemnity policies may have gaps around technology use (RCN, 2023).

Questions to ask your insurer:

Does coverage extend to claims arising from use of AI clinical decision support tools? Some policies written before AI became common may not explicitly address algorithmic recommendations. Ensure your coverage includes technology-assisted clinical decisions.

Are there exclusions for specific AI applications? Some insurers exclude experimental or inadequately validated tools. If your trust implements cutting-edge AI, verify your coverage applies.

What documentation is required to support claims? Insurers may require specific evidence showing you exercised appropriate oversight of algorithmic recommendations. Understand documentation standards expected by your insurer.

Does coverage apply if you override algorithmic recommendations? Some nurses worry that disagreeing with AI tools exposes them to liability. Good indemnity coverage should protect you for exercising clinical judgment, including when that means overriding algorithms.

Are there coverage limits specific to AI? Some policies may have lower maximum payouts for technology-related claims versus traditional clinical negligence. Ensure coverage limits are adequate.

The Royal College of Nursing provides indemnity coverage for members, including technology-related claims. But RCN guidance emphasizes that coverage depends on nurses practicing within their competence, seeking appropriate training, and exercising professional judgment rather than blindly following algorithmic recommendations (RCN, 2023).

Unison and other unions offering professional indemnity similarly cover AI-related claims but expect members to document decision-making thoroughly and demonstrate they fulfilled professional responsibilities.

What insurers won't cover:

Reckless practice: Using AI tools you're not trained to use, ignoring obvious algorithmic errors, or failing to exercise any independent judgment.

Criminal conduct: Deliberately falsifying documentation about AI use or intentionally ignoring patient safety.

Working outside scope of practice: Using AI tools requiring skills or knowledge beyond your competence without appropriate supervision.

Failing to disclose material facts: Not informing insurers about AI tools you use or claims arising from their use.

Practical steps for protection:

Inform your insurer about AI tools you use: Provide details about what systems your trust has implemented and how you use them clinically. Don't assume coverage automatically extends to new technologies.

Document thoroughly: As discussed in section 11.2, clear documentation of AI involvement in clinical decisions and your independent reasoning protects you legally and professionally.

Seek training: Ensure you receive adequate training on any AI tools you're expected to use. Document training completion. If training is insufficient, raise concerns formally.

Follow professional guidelines: Adhere to NMC standards on accountability, informed consent, record-keeping, and working within competence. These form the foundation of defensible practice.

Report concerns: If you believe AI tools are unsafe or being implemented inappropriately, raise concerns through appropriate channels. Document that you raised concerns. Whistleblowing protection applies if you report patient safety issues in good faith.

11.4 NMC Position

The Nursing and Midwifery Council regulates nursing practice in the UK, including technology use. The Code—NMC's standards of practice and behavior—applies fully to AI-augmented care (NMC, 2023).

Relevant Code requirements:

Prioritize people: "Make their care and safety your main concern, and make sure that their dignity is preserved and their needs are recognized, assessed and responded to." This means AI tools must serve patient interests, not replace careful assessment or substitute for appropriate care.

Practice effectively: "Always practice in line with the best available evidence." This requires evaluating whether AI tools you use have adequate evidence supporting their effectiveness and safety. You can't simply assume algorithmic recommendations are evidence-based without checking.

Preserve safety: "Recognize and work within the limits of your competence." If you lack training or understanding of AI tools you're expected to use, you must seek training or decline to use them. You can't claim competence you don't have.

Promote professionalism and trust: "Uphold the reputation of your profession at all times." This includes being honest about AI limitations, ensuring informed consent for algorithmic decision-making, and protecting patient confidentiality when using digital tools.

NMC's position on accountability is clear: nurses remain professionally accountable for all decisions and care they provide, including when technology is involved. AI recommendations don't transfer accountability from nurses to machines. You're responsible for evaluating algorithmic outputs and deciding whether to follow them (NMC, 2023).

Future directions for NMC guidance on AI are uncertain. The regulator is developing more specific standards for technology use in nursing but hasn't yet published comprehensive AI guidance. Expect updates as AI becomes more prevalent and regulatory gaps become apparent.

What NMC is likely to emphasize:

Informed consent: Patients must understand when AI influences their care and have opportunities to ask questions or refuse.

Clinical judgment: Nurses must exercise independent professional judgment, not defer to algorithms uncritically.

Competence: Nurses must receive adequate training on AI tools and only use them within their competence.

Documentation: Clear, accurate, contemporaneous records showing how AI influenced clinical decisions.

Patient safety: AI tools must be implemented with robust governance, monitoring, and mechanisms for identifying and addressing errors.

Nurses who follow these principles—exercising judgment, documenting thoroughly, practicing within competence, prioritizing patient safety—will generally be supported by the NMC even when outcomes are poor. Those who blindly follow flawed algorithms or use tools they don't understand will struggle to justify their practice professionally (NMC, 2023).

11.5 Protecting Yourself

Practical risk mitigation for nurses using AI:

Understand how AI tools you use actually work: Don't use systems you can't explain. If you don't know what data an algorithm uses, how it calculates risk scores, or what its limitations are, you can't use it safely.

Treat AI as advisory, never definitive: Algorithmic recommendations inform your decisions; they don't make them. Always conduct independent assessment and reach your own clinical conclusions.

Document your thinking: When following AI recommendations, note that you independently assessed the patient and agreed with the algorithmic output. When overriding AI, clearly document your clinical reasoning.

Raise concerns formally: If AI tools seem inaccurate, biased, or poorly implemented, report concerns through appropriate channels.

Written reports to managers, incident reporting systems, or clinical governance committees create records showing you identified problems.

Stay within competence: If you're asked to use AI tools you're not trained for, seek training before using them clinically. Document training completion. If adequate training isn't provided, formally document that you lack competence to use the tools safely.

Maintain therapeutic relationship: Don't let technology interfere with building rapport and understanding patients. AI provides data points; relationships provide context and trust essential for safe care.

Know your limits: There will be clinical situations where AI recommendations don't make sense. Trust your judgment. It's better to override a flawed algorithm than follow it into error.

The accountability landscape will continue evolving as AI becomes more prevalent and legal cases establish precedents. But fundamental principles won't change: you remain professionally responsible for patient care, you must exercise independent clinical judgment, and thorough documentation protects you when outcomes are poor.

Chapter 12.0: The Future Ahead

Mental health nursing won't disappear in an AI world. But it will change—perhaps profoundly. Some tasks you do now will be automated. New responsibilities will emerge. The skills that matter most will shift. And you'll need to position yourself not just as an AI user but as an advocate shaping how these technologies develop and deploy in mental health services.

The future isn't predetermined. Technology companies and policymakers are making choices now that will define mental health care for decades. Nurses can influence those choices—or be sidelined while others decide how your profession evolves. This chapter explores what's coming, which skills will remain uniquely human, how the CPN role is evolving, and what you can do to stay relevant and influential in an AI-augmented mental health system.

12.1 Irreplaceable Human Skills

What AI cannot do—at least not in foreseeable future—defines the irreplaceable core of mental health nursing:

Therapeutic presence: Being fully present with another person in their suffering, witnessing their pain without trying to fix it immediately, holding hope when they can't. Algorithms can't do this. They can process information and offer suggestions, but they can't *be with* someone in the way humans can (Topol, 2019).

Therapeutic relationship: The alliance between nurse and patient—built on trust, consistency, mutual respect, and genuine care—remains central to effective mental health care. No chatbot, however sophisticated, creates the kind of relationship where someone feels truly seen, understood, and valued as a person rather than a collection of symptoms (Horvath et al., 2011).

Contextual understanding: You understand that someone's "non-compliance" with medication might reflect inability to afford prescriptions, or cultural beliefs about medication, or past trauma with forced treatment. AI sees missed doses; you see the human story behind the pattern. That contextual understanding—requiring empathy, cultural competence, and willingness to understand rather than judge—is uniquely human.

Ethical reasoning: When algorithmic recommendations conflict with patient preferences, when resource constraints force difficult triage decisions, when advocacy might conflict with institutional priorities—these require ethical reasoning that AI cannot provide. Algorithms can optimize for defined objectives but can't grapple with values conflicts requiring human judgment (Char et al., 2018).

Creative problem-solving: Mental health recovery rarely follows linear paths. You improvise, adapt, try novel approaches when standard interventions don't work. You connect patients to unexpected resources—a community garden program, a peer support group, a vocational training opportunity—based on understanding the individual rather than following protocols. AI optimizes within parameters; humans innovate beyond them.

Advocacy: Challenging systems that harm patients, fighting for resources and rights, speaking up against discrimination—these require moral courage and political engagement that algorithms cannot provide. Your role as patient advocate is fundamentally human work (Topol, 2019).

Cultural competence: Understanding how cultural background shapes mental health experiences, symptom expression, help-seeking, family involvement, and recovery requires cultural humility and ongoing learning that AI cannot replicate. Even "culturally sensitive" algorithms are crude approximations of genuine cultural understanding.

Crisis management: Real crisis response—talking someone through acute suicidal ideation, de-escalating agitation, making split-second safety decisions—requires human judgment, flexibility, and capacity to build rapid rapport that AI cannot match. Chatbots directing people to crisis lines aren't crisis intervention; they're triage (Torous et al., 2020).

These skills won't become obsolete. They'll become more valuable as AI handles tasks that don't require human judgment, freeing you to focus on work that genuinely needs your expertise. The future of mental health nursing isn't less human—it's more human, with technology handling the tasks that distracted from therapeutic work.

12.2 The Evolving CPN

The community psychiatric nurse role is already changing. Traditional case management—coordinating appointments, monitoring medication, conducting regular reviews—is being supplemented by new responsibilities:

Care orchestration: Instead of providing all care directly, you're increasingly coordinating care across multiple providers—GPs, digital therapeutics, peer support, voluntary sector services, social care. You become the conductor ensuring all these elements work together coherently rather than the solo performer doing everything yourself (Topol, 2019).

Digital intervention management: Prescribing and monitoring digital therapeutics, troubleshooting when patients struggle with apps, integrating app-generated data into care planning, adjusting digital interventions based on response. This requires new skills—comfort with technology, ability to evaluate digital tools critically, competence explaining AI concepts to patients.

Algorithm oversight: Reviewing AI-generated risk assessments, challenging algorithmic recommendations that don't match clinical reality, providing feedback to improve system performance, advocating for patients when algorithms fail them. You're the human safeguard ensuring AI serves rather than harms patients.

Data interpretation: Making sense of digital phenotyping data, wearable sensor information, or patient-generated health data from apps and tracking tools. Understanding what patterns mean clinically, distinguishing signal from noise, explaining findings to patients in accessible language.

Technology teaching: Helping patients use digital mental health tools effectively, troubleshooting technical problems, coaching people through initial discomfort with technology-mediated care. You're part therapist, part IT support.

Systems advocacy: Identifying where AI implementations disadvantage certain populations, documenting bias, pushing for equitable tool development, ensuring clinical workflows accommodate rather than exploit technology. You're advocating not just for individual patients but for system-level fairness.

The shift is from direct care provider to care coordinator, from primary relationship to relationship facilitator, from doing everything yourself to orchestrating various elements—human and technological—that contribute to recovery. Some nurses embrace this evolution; others mourn the loss of what felt like more authentic therapeutic work (Topol, 2019).

There's room for both approaches. Mental health nursing is diversifying—some roles will involve heavy AI integration and technology orchestration, while others maintain more traditional therapeutic focus. Your career path can reflect your preferences and strengths. But understanding the direction of change helps you prepare rather than being caught off-guard.

12.3 Next Wave Technologies

What's coming beyond current AI applications:

Virtual reality therapy: Immersive VR environments for exposure therapy (treating phobias, PTSD, anxiety), skills practice (social skills training, job interview preparation), and experiential interventions (mindfulness, relaxation, perspective-taking). Early evidence shows effectiveness comparable to traditional exposure therapy, with potential advantages in safety, consistency, and accessibility (Freeman et al., 2017).

Nurses might deliver VR-assisted therapy, guiding patients through virtual exposures while monitoring anxiety responses and providing in-session support. Or you might prescribe VR programs for home use, similar to how you might prescribe DTx apps now.

Predictive genomics: Genetic testing to predict which medications will work best for which patients, personalized risk assessment based on genetic markers, and targeted interventions based on biological profiles. The field is still emerging, with significant ethical concerns about privacy, discrimination, and reductionism (Roberts et al., 2021).

Your role might include explaining genetic testing to patients, helping them interpret results, and integrating genetic information into care planning—all while being skeptical about overstated claims from companies selling genetic testing services.

Brain-computer interfaces: Direct neural monitoring and stimulation for treatment-resistant depression, anxiety, or psychosis. Early-stage research shows promise but raises profound questions about autonomy, identity, and risks of unintended effects (Yuste et al., 2017).

You probably won't be implanting electrodes in patients' brains, but you might monitor patients using neurostimulation devices, assess response, and provide psychosocial support addressing the psychological impact of brain-interfacing technology.

Ambient sensors: Home-based monitoring systems detecting changes in speech patterns, movement, social interaction, or physiological markers indicating deteriorating mental health. Think of it as digital phenotyping on steroids—passive monitoring across multiple data streams creating comprehensive behavioral profiles (Torous et al., 2020).

Ethical concerns about surveillance, privacy, and autonomy are substantial. But if implemented with appropriate safeguards, such systems might enable earlier intervention and reduce crisis admissions. Your role: explaining systems to patients, interpreting data, ensuring monitoring serves therapeutic goals rather than just institutional risk management.

AI-generated personalized content: Therapeutic interventions, psychoeducation materials, coping skills training, and relapse prevention plans automatically generated and tailored to individual patient characteristics. Instead of giving everyone the same CBT workbook, AI creates customized materials reflecting the person's specific symptoms, cultural background, literacy level, and treatment goals (Torous et al., 2020).

You'd review AI-generated materials for appropriateness, modify them based on clinical judgment, and use them as springboards for therapeutic conversations rather than replacements for them.

Social media monitoring: Algorithms analyzing public social media posts to identify mental health deterioration, crisis risk, or treatment response. Already happening in research settings; likely to expand despite significant privacy and ethical concerns (Ernala et al., 2019).

Should mental health services monitor patients' social media for warning signs? Some patients might welcome it as protective; others would find it invasive and creepy. Navigating these tensions will require careful ethical reasoning and genuine patient involvement in deciding what's acceptable.

12.4 Nurse Led Development

AI development has been dominated by computer scientists, engineers, and data scientists with limited clinical expertise and minimal input from frontline staff. This creates tools that are technically sophisticated but clinically impractical, workflows that disrupt rather than enhance care, and algorithms that don't reflect what actually matters to patients and practitioners (Shaw et al., 2019).

Nurses need to be at the table during AI development, not just asked to implement what others designed. Your expertise is essential for:

Identifying problems worth solving: Developers don't know which tasks consume your time unproductively, which clinical challenges lack good solutions, which patient populations are underserved. You do. Nurse-led problem identification ensures AI addresses real needs rather than problems developers imagine.

Designing practical workflows: Algorithms that require five clicks, three screen transitions, and duplicate data entry won't get used. Nurses understand workflow realities in ways developers cannot. Your input during design prevents creation of technically brilliant tools that are practically useless (Shaw et al., 2019).

Defining success meaningfully: Developers optimize for metrics they can measure—accuracy rates, computational efficiency, processing speed. You know that success means patients feeling better, staff having sustainable workloads, and care feeling human despite technological mediation. These outcomes are harder to quantify but more important.

Ensuring ethical implementation: Nurses bring perspectives on patient autonomy, dignity, equity, and justice that purely technical development teams often miss. Your ethical expertise helps prevent AI deployments that are technically functional but ethically problematic.

Providing lived experience: Many mental health nurses have personal experience with mental illness—either their own or that of loved ones. This lived experience offers insights into what patients need, how interventions land emotionally, and what matters beyond symptom reduction. Development teams lacking this perspective create tools that feel detached from human reality.

How to get involved:

Join AI development teams: Some trusts and universities have projects developing mental health AI and need clinical expertise. Volunteer. Make it clear you bring essential knowledge they're missing.

Participate in co-design: User-centered design methodologies involve end users—including clinicians and patients—throughout development. Participate in workshops, provide feedback on prototypes, test early versions, and demand changes when tools don't work.

Partner with researchers: Academic researchers developing mental health AI often seek clinical collaborators. Contact researchers at universities doing relevant work and offer your expertise.

Advocate for nursing leadership: Push for nurses to hold leadership positions in digital health transformation, not just staff-level roles. Nurses leading AI strategy ensures clinical priorities shape development.

Pursue additional education: Programs in health informatics, digital health, or health data science with clinical backgrounds are emerging. These prepare nurses for leadership roles in AI development and implementation (Topol, 2019).

Write and speak: Publish about your experiences with AI in clinical practice—what works, what fails, what patients need. Speak at conferences, contribute to professional forums, and make nursing perspectives visible in AI discussions.

Advocate for funding: AI development for corporate profit gets substantial investment; AI development serving patient and clinician needs gets far less. Advocate for public investment in health AI that prioritizes clinical benefit over profit.

Maria, a nurse practitioner with interest in digital health (composite example), noticed that AI triage tools consistently misclassified patients experiencing dissociation or PTSD-related symptoms. She documented patterns, reached out to the tool's developers, and offered to collaborate on improvements. The company welcomed her input—they hadn't anticipated these failure modes. Maria's clinical expertise led to algorithm modifications that improved accuracy for trauma presentations. That's the impact nurses can have when we engage with rather than just endure AI development.

12.5 Staying Relevant

Continuous learning is essential in a rapidly changing field. The AI tools you learn about today will be outdated in five years. The skills valued now may shift. Staying ahead requires ongoing investment in professional development.

Practical strategies:

Follow digital health news: Subscribe to journals like *JMIR Mental Health, Digital Psychiatry, NPJ Digital Medicine*. Follow thought leaders in digital mental health on social media. Stay informed about emerging technologies and evidence.

Attend conferences: Digital health tracks at nursing conferences, specialized digital mental health conferences, and interdisciplinary meetings bring you into contact with innovators and expose you to cutting-edge developments.

Network with innovators: Connect with colleagues working on digital health projects, researchers studying AI in mental health, and developers creating tools. Conversations with people doing innovative work keep you informed and create collaboration opportunities.

Seek training: Formal courses in health informatics, data literacy, digital therapeutics, or AI in healthcare are increasingly available. Many are online, part-time, and designed for working clinicians (Topol, 2019).

Experiment with tools: Download and try mental health apps, play with AI chatbots, explore digital therapeutics. Personal experience helps you understand what patients encounter and evaluate tools more critically.

Read beyond nursing: Computer science, ethics, sociology, and policy literature on AI offers perspectives missing from clinical publications. Interdisciplinary reading makes you a more sophisticated AI user and critic.

Develop specialized expertise: Become the digital health expert in your team or service. Specialization makes you valuable, creates career opportunities, and ensures you're consulted when AI implementations occur.

Teach others: Leading training on digital therapeutics, presenting on AI in mental health, or mentoring colleagues interested in technology solidifies your expertise and positions you as a leader.

Stay skeptical: Not every AI innovation is beneficial. Critical evaluation—distinguishing genuine advances from hyped rubbish—is a skill worth cultivating. Read methodology sections of studies, demand evidence, question claims, and maintain healthy skepticism about corporate promises.

The future of mental health nursing will be shaped by those who engage with rather than resist technological change. That doesn't mean uncritical acceptance of everything marketed as innovation. It means thoughtful engagement—understanding technology deeply enough to use it well, recognize its limitations, and advocate for developments that genuinely serve patients.

You have a choice: be passive consumers of technologies others create, or active participants shaping how AI develops and deploys in mental health care. The latter is far more interesting, professionally rewarding, and beneficial for patients. The tools are here. The question is whether nurses will lead the way forward or follow paths others define.

Chapter 13.0: Getting Started Today

You've read about AI in mental health nursing. You understand the opportunities and risks. You're convinced that integrating AI thoughtfully could improve your practice and patient outcomes. Now what?

The gap between understanding AI conceptually and actually implementing it in clinical practice is substantial. Most nurses want to use AI effectively but don't know where to start. Should you experiment with every new app? Wait for your trust to mandate tools? Focus on one application area? The abundance of choices creates paralysis.

This chapter provides a concrete 90-day roadmap for integrating AI into your mental health nursing practice. Not theoretical principles—actual steps you can take starting today. By the end of 90 days, you'll have identified opportunities, piloted at least one AI tool, evaluated its effectiveness, and made informed decisions about scaling or pivoting. You'll also know how to build support from colleagues and management for broader AI adoption.

13.1 Days One Through Thirty

The first month focuses on assessment. You can't improve what you don't understand, so begin by mapping your current workflow, identifying pain points, and determining where AI might actually help rather than just adding complexity (Shaw et al., 2019).

Week 1: Workflow Documentation

Spend one week documenting everything you do. Create a simple log capturing:

- Clinical activities (assessments, interventions, documentation)
- Time spent on each activity
- Administrative tasks (scheduling, care coordination, paperwork)
- Frustration points (tasks that feel inefficient or redundant)
- Information gaps (decisions where you wish you had better data)

Don't change your behavior during this week—just observe and record. The goal is understanding your baseline reality, not performing an idealized version of your work.

Elena, a CPN working in community mental health (composite example), tracked her time for a week and discovered she spent 12 hours on documentation, 8 hours on care coordination phone calls, 15 hours in direct patient contact, and 5 hours in meetings. Her biggest frustration was chasing information from other services—GPs, social care, housing support—to understand the full picture of patients' circumstances. She identified care coordination as her primary pain point.

Week 2: AI Opportunity Mapping

Review your workflow documentation and ask: Where could AI realistically help? Focus on tasks that are:

- **Time-consuming but routine**: Scheduling, documentation, information gathering
- **Pattern recognition dependent**: Risk assessment, symptom tracking, treatment response prediction
- **Resource intensive**: Monitoring between appointments, providing 24/7 support access
- **Currently inadequate**: Connecting patients to community resources, tracking outcomes systematically

For each identified opportunity, note:

- Current time/resource investment
- Quality of current approach (what's working, what's not)
- Potential AI applications (triage algorithms, chatbots, digital phenotyping, etc.)
- Barriers to implementation (technical skills, cost, organizational support)

Marcus, another CPN (composite example), identified three opportunities: reducing time spent on intake paperwork through automated data collection, improving risk monitoring between monthly appointments using mood tracking apps, and connecting patients to peer support through AI-matched online communities. He prioritized the middle option as most impactful for patient safety.

Week 3: Research Available Tools

Investigate AI tools relevant to your identified opportunities. Look for:

- **Evidence base**: Published research showing effectiveness
- **Regulatory status**: NICE approval, MHRA certification, NHS Digital endorsement
- **User reviews**: What do other clinicians and patients say?
- **Implementation requirements**: Technical infrastructure, training needs, cost
- **Data governance**: Privacy protections, data ownership, security measures

Create a comparison spreadsheet for each tool category you're considering. Don't just accept marketing claims—dig into actual evidence and user experiences (Torous et al., 2020).

Resources for tool research:

- NICE Evidence Search for digital health technologies
- NHS Apps Library for approved applications
- ORCHA (Organisation for the Review of Care and Health Apps) ratings

- Published reviews in journals like *JMIR Mental Health*
- Professional networks and colleagues' experiences

Week 4: Stakeholder Consultation

Before proceeding, consult key stakeholders:

- **Patients**: What are their technology comfort levels? What kinds of digital support would they value? What are their privacy concerns?
- **Colleagues**: Who's already experimenting with AI? What's worked and what hasn't? Who might join you in piloting tools?
- **Management**: What are organizational priorities around digital health? What approval processes exist for new tools? What budget might be available?
- **IT and information governance**: What technical requirements and data protection standards must be met?

James (composite example) conducted an informal survey with 20 patients on his caseload, finding that 85% owned smartphones, 60% already used health apps, and most were open to digital mental health tools if they supplemented rather than replaced face-to-face care. This data proved valuable later when building his business case.

13.2 Days Thirty One Through Sixty

Month two is implementation. You've identified opportunities and researched options—now pilot one AI tool in a controlled, systematic way that allows meaningful evaluation (Shaw et al., 2019).

Selecting Your Pilot Tool

Choose based on:

- **Clear value proposition**: Addresses a real problem you documented in month one
- **Manageable scope**: Something you can pilot with 10-20 patients over 4-6 weeks
- **Available support**: Vendor training, colleague expertise, or clear documentation
- **Low barriers**: Minimal cost, simple implementation, compatible with existing systems
- **Measurement potential**: You can track whether it's actually helping

Avoid picking the flashiest or most cutting-edge tool. Choose something practical with proven effectiveness that solves a real problem.

Implementation Checklist

Complete these steps before launching your pilot:

Technical preparation:

- [ ] Tool installed/configured correctly
- [ ] Integration with existing systems tested
- [ ] Security and data protection requirements verified
- [ ] Backup plans for technical failures established
- [ ] Your own competence with the tool confirmed

Governance and approval:

- [ ] Information governance approval obtained
- [ ] Clinical governance notification completed
- [ ] Risk assessment documented
- [ ] Professional indemnity insurer informed if required
- [ ] Management awareness and support confirmed

Patient preparation:

- [ ] Information sheets created explaining the tool

- [ ] Consent process designed and documented
- [ ] Patient selection criteria established
- [ ] Opt-out mechanisms clear and accessible

Evaluation framework:

- [ ] Baseline metrics recorded (time spent, patient outcomes, etc.)
- [ ] Success criteria defined clearly
- [ ] Data collection methods established
- [ ] Feedback mechanisms created for patients and yourself
- [ ] Timeline for evaluation decided

Support systems:

- [ ] Colleague backup identified if you need help
- [ ] Vendor support contact information accessible
- [ ] Patient troubleshooting resources prepared
- [ ] Escalation pathways for problems established

Maria (composite example) piloted a mood tracking app with 15 patients experiencing depression. She completed all checklist items, including creating a one-page patient information sheet, obtaining information governance approval, and establishing weekly check-ins to discuss app data during scheduled appointments. Her success criteria were: 80% patient engagement with daily mood logging, reduced time spent on symptom assessment in appointments, and at least 60% of patients finding the tool helpful.

Week 5-8: Active Pilot

During the pilot:

- **Meet patients where they are**: Some will embrace technology easily; others need more support. Adjust your approach individually.

- **Expect technical problems**: Apps crash, data doesn't sync, patients forget passwords. Have troubleshooting protocols ready.
- **Stay flexible**: If something isn't working, adapt quickly rather than rigidly following your initial plan.
- **Document everything**: Record successes, failures, unexpected benefits, unanticipated problems, patient feedback, and your own observations.
- **Communicate regularly**: Keep colleagues, management, and patients informed about how the pilot is progressing.

Common pilot challenges and solutions:

Challenge: Patients don't engage consistently with the tool. **Solution**: Explore barriers. Is it too complicated? Do they forget? Is it not valuable to them? Adjust onboarding, send reminders, or reconsider whether the tool fits their needs.

Challenge: Data quality is poor (incomplete, inaccurate, not useful). **Solution**: Improve training on how to use the tool properly, simplify what you're asking patients to track, or consider whether the tool design is fundamentally problematic.

Challenge: Integration with existing workflow is clunky. **Solution**: Redesign how you're incorporating the tool. Maybe you're trying to use it in ways that don't fit naturally. Find simpler integration points.

Challenge: You're spending more time, not less. **Solution**: This is common in early implementation. Decide whether time investment will decrease as you gain proficiency, or whether the tool genuinely isn't efficient.

13.3 Days Sixty One Through Ninety

Month three is evaluation and decision-making. You've piloted a tool for 4-6 weeks—now determine whether to scale it, modify it, or abandon it (Greenhalgh et al., 2017).

Systematic Evaluation

Review your predefined success criteria against actual outcomes:

Quantitative metrics:

- Time saved or added to your workflow
- Patient engagement rates (how many used the tool as intended?)
- Clinical outcomes (symptom improvement, crisis rates, appointment attendance)
- Cost (actual expenses versus budgeted)
- Technical reliability (uptime, errors, data loss incidents)

Qualitative feedback:

- Patient satisfaction and perceived usefulness
- Your own experience using the tool
- Colleague observations
- Unexpected benefits or problems
- Scalability concerns

Aisha (composite example) evaluated her digital phenotyping pilot with 12 patients. Quantitatively, 75% engaged consistently, she detected deterioration 5-7 days earlier than usual in three cases, and she spent an extra 30 minutes weekly reviewing data. Qualitatively, patients appreciated feeling monitored between appointments but several found the passive tracking slightly creepy. She felt the early warning benefit justified continued use but needed better patient education about privacy.

Decision Framework

Based on evaluation, choose one of three paths:

Scale: Tool worked well enough to expand to more patients or colleagues. This doesn't mean perfection—just clear net benefit and manageable problems.

Iterate: Tool shows promise but needs modifications before broader implementation. Maybe you need different patient selection criteria, better training materials, workflow adjustments, or vendor improvements.

Pivot: Tool didn't deliver expected value, created more problems than it solved, or patients/you didn't find it useful. Abandon this approach and try something different. This isn't failure—it's learning (Greenhalgh et al., 2017).

If scaling, create an implementation plan:

- How many additional patients over what timeframe?
- What resources are needed (training, licenses, support)?
- Who else on your team will be involved?
- How will you maintain quality as you expand?
- What ongoing evaluation will occur?

If iterating, specify what needs to change:

- Particular features causing problems
- Training improvements needed
- Workflow redesign required
- Patient population adjustments
- Timeline for next pilot round

If pivoting, document lessons learned:

- Why didn't this work?
- What would you do differently next time?
- Are there other tools worth trying for the same problem?
- Should you focus on a different problem entirely?

13.4 Building Management Support

Most AI implementation requires organizational support—budget, technical infrastructure, information governance approval, training resources. Building a compelling business case increases your chances of securing that support (Shaw et al., 2019).

Elements of an effective business case:

Problem definition: What specific problem are you addressing? Use data from your workflow audit showing time spent, resources consumed, gaps in care, or adverse outcomes. Make the problem concrete and quantifiable.

Example: "Our service has 450 referrals waiting over 8 weeks for initial assessment. Current triage relies on GP referral letters providing limited information. Clinicians spend 60-90 minutes per initial assessment gathering information that could be collected digitally beforehand. This creates bottlenecks reducing access to care."

Proposed solution: Which AI tool addresses the problem and how? Include evidence of effectiveness from published research, other NHS implementations, or your pilot data if available (Torous & Roberts, 2017).

Example: "An AI-powered digital intake tool collects patient-reported symptoms, history, and preferences before initial appointments. NICE-approved system used by 15 other NHS trusts. Published research shows 40% reduction in assessment time while improving data quality. Our 60-day pilot with 20 patients reduced initial assessment from 75 to 45 minutes while capturing more comprehensive information."

Benefits: What improvements will occur? Consider multiple benefit categories:

Patient benefits:

- Faster access to care
- More personalized treatment
- Better outcomes

- Improved satisfaction
- Reduced crisis episodes

Clinician benefits:

- Time saved on administrative tasks
- Better information for decision-making
- Reduced burnout
- Ability to manage larger caseloads safely

Organizational benefits:

- Improved efficiency and throughput
- Cost savings or cost avoidance
- Better quality metrics
- Reduced adverse events
- Enhanced reputation

Quantify benefits wherever possible using your pilot data or published evidence.

Costs: Be honest about all costs involved:

- Initial licensing or purchase
- Ongoing subscription fees
- Implementation time and training
- Technical infrastructure requirements
- Maintenance and support
- Evaluation and quality assurance

Include both financial costs and time costs (which ultimately are financial costs to the organization).

Implementation plan: How will this actually happen?

- Timeline with specific milestones
- Roles and responsibilities
- Training requirements

- Technical prerequisites
- Risk mitigation strategies
- Evaluation measures

Risk assessment: What could go wrong and how will you mitigate those risks?

- Technical failures (backup systems, vendor support agreements)
- Poor patient engagement (thorough training, ongoing support)
- Inadequate data quality (validation processes, quality checks)
- Privacy breaches (robust security measures, regular audits)
- Clinical errors (human oversight requirements, clear limitations)

Presentation tips:

Lead with impact: Start with the patient or organizational problem you're solving, not the technology itself. Decision-makers care about outcomes, not features.

Use stories and data: Combine compelling patient examples (anonymized) with quantitative evidence. Stories create emotional engagement; data proves viability.

Address concerns proactively: Anticipate objections (cost, technical complexity, staff resistance, patient privacy) and address them directly in your proposal.

Show momentum: If you've already piloted successfully, emphasize that. If other services are using similar tools, note that. Reduce perceived risk by showing this isn't experimental.

Be realistic about limitations: Don't oversell. Acknowledge that AI won't solve everything, implementation will be challenging, and success isn't guaranteed. Credibility matters more than salesmanship.

Diego (composite example) built a business case for digital therapeutics apps to supplement face-to-face CBT sessions. His proposal showed that delivering 6 face-to-face sessions plus app-based exercises produced similar outcomes to 12 face-to-face sessions in published research, potentially doubling therapist capacity. He included pilot data from 10 patients, cost analysis showing break-even at 18 months, and testimonials from patients who found the apps helpful. Management approved a 6-month expansion trial with 50 patients.

13.5 Creating Champion Networks

Individual enthusiasm hits limits quickly. Sustainable AI integration requires building a network of colleagues who understand, support, and actively use these tools (Greenhalgh et al., 2017).

Identifying potential champions:

Look for colleagues who:

- Express curiosity about digital health
- Are early adopters of technology generally
- Feel frustrated by inefficiencies AI might address
- Have influence in your organization (formal or informal)
- Are respected by peers for clinical judgment
- Value innovation but maintain healthy skepticism

Don't assume champions will be young or tech-savvy. Some of the best digital health advocates are experienced clinicians who recognize how technology can solve problems they've struggled with for years.

Recruitment strategies:

Share your experiences: Talk about what you're learning, both successes and failures. Authenticity builds trust. Colleagues are more likely to engage when they see someone like them navigating AI practically rather than evangelizing theoretically.

Provide hands-on exposure: Invite colleagues to observe your use of AI tools, try them briefly with their own patients (if appropriate), or review your pilot data. Direct experience is more persuasive than descriptions.

Address concerns directly: Many nurses have legitimate worries about AI—job displacement, dehumanization of care, privacy risks, inadequate training. Don't dismiss these concerns. Acknowledge them and discuss how thoughtful implementation mitigates risks.

Start small: Don't ask colleagues to overhaul their entire practice. Invite them to try one tool with a few patients for a few weeks. Lower the barrier to entry.

Provide support: Offer to help with setup, troubleshooting, patient education, or documentation. Make it as easy as possible for colleagues to experiment.

Network activities:

Regular meetings: Monthly gatherings (formal or informal) to share experiences, troubleshoot problems, discuss new tools, and support each other's learning. Virtual meetings work if colleagues are geographically dispersed.

Shared resources: Collaborative documents containing tool reviews, patient information sheets, implementation checklists, evaluation templates, and lessons learned. Build institutional knowledge collectively (Shaw et al., 2019).

Peer learning sessions: Colleagues teaching each other about tools they've mastered, challenges they've overcome, or workflows they've designed. Peer learning is often more credible than external training.

Pilot collaborations: Multiple champions piloting the same tool simultaneously allows comparison of approaches, pooling of data for stronger evaluation, and mutual support through challenges.

Advocacy coordination: When seeking organizational support, a network can present unified proposals, share the workload of business case development, and demonstrate broader enthusiasm than individual requests convey.

Management engagement: Champion networks have more leverage than individuals to influence digital health strategy, participate in procurement decisions, and shape implementation policies.

Nicole created a "Digital Mental Health Nurses" group (composite example) with seven colleagues across her trust. They met monthly over lunch, shared a Google Drive folder with resources, piloted different apps and compared notes, and collectively proposed an AI triage system to management—which was approved partly because the proposal demonstrated multi-clinician support rather than one person's pet project.

13.6 Moving Forward

Ninety days from today, you could be using AI tools that improve your practice, save time, or enhance patient outcomes. Or you could still be thinking about it theoretically while the gap between early adopters and late adopters widens. The difference isn't intelligence or resources—it's starting.

Choose one small thing to do today. Document your workflow for a week. Research one AI tool category. Talk to one colleague about their digital health experiments. Each small action builds momentum toward meaningful integration.

The roadmap in this chapter isn't prescriptive—adapt it to your circumstances, your service, your patient population, and your organizational culture. But the fundamental process applies universally: assess, pilot, evaluate, decide, build support, and create sustainable networks. That's how individual enthusiasm becomes organizational transformation.

Chapter 14.0: Resources and Next Steps

You've reached the end of this textbook, but you're just beginning your journey with AI in mental health nursing. The field changes rapidly—new tools emerge, research evolves, regulations shift, and best practices develop through collective experience. Staying current requires knowing where to find reliable information, which courses build relevant skills, which professional networks support continued learning, and how to maintain critical perspective as the AI hype cycle continues (Topol, 2019).

This chapter provides concrete resources for deepening your expertise. Not comprehensive listings of everything available—those would be outdated before publication—but curated starting points for high-quality education, vetted tools, active professional communities, and strategies for lifelong learning in this rapidly evolving field.

14.1 Education and Training

Formal courses and certifications provide structured learning, recognized credentials, and often access to expert instructors and peer networks. Several programs specifically target healthcare professionals seeking AI and digital health competence (Topol, 2019).

NHS Digital Academy: The Academy's digital health leadership programs prepare senior nurses and other clinicians for strategic roles in healthcare technology. The **Digital Health Leadership Programme** is a year-long course combining online learning, in-person workshops, and practical projects. Participants learn health informatics, AI basics, change management, and digital transformation strategy. Open to Band 7+ nurses with demonstrated leadership potential. NHS organizations typically sponsor participants. Details at https://www.hee.nhs.uk/our-work/digital-health-leadership

Strengths: NHS-specific context, strong networking opportunities, organizational recognition of credentials, no direct cost to participants.

Limitations: Competitive application process, requires significant time commitment, focused on leadership rather than hands-on clinical AI skills.

Royal College of Nursing Digital Health Resources: The RCN provides various learning materials on digital health, though not comprehensive AI training. Their website includes guidance documents, webinars, and position statements on technology in nursing. Members can access recorded sessions from past conferences covering digital health topics. Useful for understanding professional context and regulatory expectations more than technical skills. Resources at https://www.rcn.org.uk/clinical-topics/digital-health

Strengths: Free for RCN members, nursing-specific perspective, regularly updated.

Limitations: Not comprehensive AI education, limited depth on technical topics, variable quality across resources.

Health Education England (HEE) Digital Literacy Framework: HEE's framework defines digital capabilities expected of healthcare staff at different levels. Useful for self-assessment and identifying learning needs. The framework covers digital identity and wellbeing, information and data literacy, communication and collaboration, teaching and learning, technical proficiency, and creation and innovation. Available at https://www.hee.nhs.uk/our-work/digital-literacy

Strengths: Provides clear competency standards, useful for professional development planning, widely recognized in NHS.

Limitations: Framework describes competencies but doesn't teach them, requires seeking separate learning resources for skill development.

University-Based Programs:

Several UK universities offer postgraduate certificates, diplomas, or Master's programs in health informatics, digital health, or health data science that include AI components:

University College London (UCL): MSc in Digital Health offers modules on AI in healthcare, data analytics, and digital therapeutics. Part-time online study available for working professionals.

Imperial College London: MSc in Health Data Analytics and Machine Learning teaches statistical and machine learning methods applied to health data. Requires quantitative background.

University of Edinburgh: MSc in Clinical Artificial Intelligence combines clinical and technical training. Designed for healthcare professionals wanting to develop AI systems.

King's College London: MSc in Digital Health & Entrepreneurship covers technology development and implementation in health

care settings, including AI applications.

These programs vary substantially in technical depth, time commitment, cost, and required prerequisites. Research carefully to ensure fit with your goals and background.

Strengths: Recognized qualifications, comprehensive learning, access to research and expert faculty, potential career advancement.

Limitations: Substantial time and financial investment, may be more technical than clinically-focused nurses need, balancing with full-time work challenging.

Online Courses and MOOCs:

Coursera, edX, FutureLearn: Multiple platforms offer courses on AI, machine learning, and digital health. Quality varies substantially. Look for courses from reputable institutions with healthcare focus.

Notable examples:

- Stanford's "Machine Learning" (Coursera) provides technical AI foundations but isn't healthcare-specific
- MIT's "Data Science for Healthcare" (edX) applies data analysis to clinical questions
- University of Michigan's "AI in Healthcare" (Coursera) covers applications specifically for clinicians

Strengths: Flexible timing, lower cost, wide variety of topics, learn at your own pace.

Limitations: Variable quality, limited interaction with instructors, no clinical context for general AI courses, less recognized than formal qualifications.

Professional Development Through Employers:

Many NHS trusts offer digital health training to staff. Check with your Learning and Development department about:

- In-house training on specific AI tools your organization implements
- Funded external courses aligned with service needs
- Time allocation for professional development
- Mentoring or shadowing opportunities with digital health leads

14.2 Vetted AI Tools

Digital therapeutics, clinical decision support systems, and patient-facing apps vary enormously in quality, evidence base, and appropriateness for NHS use. This section provides starting points for identifying trustworthy tools, not exhaustive listings (which would quickly become outdated).

NHS Apps Library (https://www.nhs.uk/apps-library/): NHS Digital's curated collection of health apps meeting minimum standards for clinical safety, data protection, and usability. Apps are assessed against the Digital Technology Assessment Criteria (DTAC). Search by condition and filter by evidence level.

Pros: NHS-endorsed, vetted for basic safety and privacy, organized by condition, free access to information.

Cons: Inclusion doesn't guarantee clinical effectiveness (only that apps aren't dangerous), quality varies substantially, limited critical review of evidence, somewhat limited selection.

ORCHA (Organisation for the Review of Care and Health Apps) (https://orchahealth.com): Independent health app evaluation service. Reviews apps against 350+ points covering clinical safety, data privacy, usability, and evidence. Generates objective scores. Some NHS trusts subscribe to ORCHA, providing staff with access to detailed reviews. Individual reviews available for fee.

Pros: Rigorous evaluation methodology, transparent scoring, covers wide range of apps, regularly updated, identifies specific strengths and weaknesses.

Cons: Subscription required for full access, high score doesn't guarantee app is right for your patient population, evaluation is technical rather than capturing lived experience.

NICE Evidence Standards Framework for Digital Health Technologies: NICE's framework describes evidence expectations for different technology categories. Useful for evaluating whether tools you're considering meet appropriate evidence standards. Framework doesn't review specific products but helps you know what questions to ask. Available at https://www.nice.org.uk/about/what-we-do/our-programmes/evidence-standards-framework-for-digital-health-technologies

Examples of Evidence-Based Mental Health AI Tools:

SilverCloud (Amwell): Online CBT and other therapeutic programs for depression, anxiety, and stress. NICE-approved for NHS use. Delivered through therapist-supported or self-directed models. Strong research base showing effectiveness comparable to face-to-face therapy for mild-moderate conditions (Richards et al., 2015).

Pros: Extensive evidence, NICE-approved, multiple conditions covered, therapist support option, used by many NHS trusts.

Cons: Subscription cost, requires consistent patient engagement, less effective for severe presentations, limited personalization.

Sleepio (Big Health): Digital CBT for insomnia. NICE-approved. Fully automated six-week program. Research shows improvements in sleep quality and duration comparable to face-to-face CBT for insomnia (Espie et al., 2019).

Pros: Strong evidence base, automated delivery (no clinician time needed), scalable, NICE-approved.

Cons: Limited to insomnia, requires patient tech comfort, dropout rates ~30-40%, cost per license.

Wysa: AI chatbot providing emotional support and CBT techniques. Uses natural language processing to simulate conversations. Less evidence than SilverCloud or Sleepio, but growing research base. Available in NHS Apps Library (Inkster et al., 2018).

Pros: Immediate 24/7 access, low cost, conversational interface feels natural to many users, covers multiple conditions.

Cons: Limited evidence compared to established DTx, concerns about accuracy of AI responses, data privacy questions in past versions, no human backup for high-risk situations.

Important caveat: Tool recommendations here aren't endorsements. Technology changes constantly. Always verify current evidence, regulatory status, and organizational approval before clinical use. What's appropriate for one patient population or service context may not suit another.

14.3 Professional Networks

Learning happens in community. Connecting with other mental health nurses exploring AI creates opportunities to share experiences, troubleshoot problems, learn about new tools, and advocate collectively for better technology (Topol, 2019).

RCN Digital Health Network: Informal network of RCN members interested in digital health. Occasional webinars, forum discussions, and conference meet-ups. Join through RCN membership website. More focused on general digital health than specifically AI, but relevant overlapping interests.

Pros: Easy access for RCN members, nursing-specific, professional credibility, free participation.

Cons: Not very active compared to other communities, limited AI-specific content, relies on volunteer organization.

DigitalHealth.London Innovation Network: Network connecting digital health innovators, clinicians, and organizations in London region. Regular events, workshops, and networking opportunities. Open to healthcare professionals interested in digital transformation. Some events are London-specific but others virtual.

Website: https://www.digitalhealth.london

Pros: Active community, access to innovators and developers, exposure to cutting-edge developments, good for staying informed about emerging tech.

Cons: London-centric, variable relevance to direct clinical practice, can feel commercial rather than clinically-focused.

AI in Health and Care Award Winners Network: The Secretary of State's annual AI Awards recognize excellent AI implementations in NHS. Winners form an informal network sharing learnings. Following award winners on social media or reaching out directly often yields generous knowledge sharing from people who've successfully implemented AI at scale.

Pros: Learn from proven implementations, evidence-based approaches, practical insights from real deployments.

Cons: Informal network without structured organization, requires individual initiative to connect.

Twitter/X and LinkedIn: Active digital health communities exist on social media. Following key thought leaders, participating in discussions, and sharing your own experiences builds networks and keeps you informed. Relevant hashtags include #DigitalHealth, #HealthcareAI, #DigitalMentalHealth, #NHSDigital.

Pros: Real-time updates, diverse international perspectives, easy access, free participation, direct engagement with experts.

Cons: Signal-to-noise ratio challenging, information quality variable, commercial interests disguised as education, can be time-consuming.

Local Trust Digital Health Groups: Many trusts have clinical technology user groups, digital transformation committees, or innovation networks. Internal networks provide immediate relevance to your service context and direct influence on local implementations. Ask your Chief Nursing Information Officer or Digital Health Lead about existing groups.

Pros: Directly relevant to your work context, potential influence on local decisions, face-to-face networking, organizational support.

Cons: Quality varies by trust, may be dominated by IT rather than clinical perspectives, internal politics can complicate advocacy.

14.4 Staying Current

The landscape shifts constantly. New research, emerging tools, regulatory updates, and evolving best practices mean that expertise requires ongoing learning rather than one-time training (Topol, 2019).

Essential Journals:

JMIR Mental Health (https://mental.jmir.org): Open-access journal specifically focused on digital mental health interventions, including AI applications. Publishes research on effectiveness, implementation, and user experiences of digital mental health tools. Monthly scanning of new issues keeps you informed about latest evidence.

NPJ Digital Medicine (https://www.nature.com/npjdigitalmed): Nature's open-access journal covering digital medicine broadly, including substantial AI content. High-quality research, rigorous peer review, covers clinical applications rather than just technical development.

The Lancet Digital Health (https://www.thelancet.com/journals/landig): Prestigious journal publishing research, reviews, and commentary on digital health innovations. Includes AI applications in mental health among broader digital health content.

British Journal of Psychiatry and **Advances in Psychiatric Treatment**: While not AI-specific, these journals increasingly publish articles on digital mental health and technology in psychiatric care relevant to nursing practice.

How to stay current without drowning: Set up table-of-contents alerts from 2-3 key journals. Scan titles monthly, read abstracts of relevant articles, deep-read 1-2 particularly applicable pieces. Quality over quantity.

Podcasts:

Digital Health on TenToTheTwenty (NHS Digital): Podcast interviewing digital health leaders about NHS technology innovations. Episodes cover AI implementations, lessons learned, and strategic thinking about technology transformation.

The Health Innovators Network: Interviews with healthcare technology innovators, including AI developers and implementing clinicians. Provides both technical understanding and practical implementation insights.

BBC's Health Check: Not specifically digital health, but regularly covers AI and technology in healthcare among broader health topics. Good for understanding public perception and media framing of health AI.

Podcasts are efficient learning tools during commutes, exercise, or household tasks—passive learning that accumulates over time without requiring dedicated study sessions.

Thought Leaders to Follow:

Dr. Eric Topol (@EricTopol): Cardiologist and researcher focusing on AI in medicine. Author of "Deep Medicine" about AI's potential to restore humanity in healthcare. Provides balanced perspective acknowledging both promise and risks. Prolific Twitter/X presence sharing latest research and thoughtful commentary.

Dr. Helen Salisbury (@HelenRSalisbury): GP writing about technology in primary care, including AI. Offers critical clinical perspective on digital health, not afraid to challenge hype.

Dr. Hugh Harvey (@DrHughHarvey): Radiologist specializing in AI, provides technical depth accessible to non-experts. Good source for understanding how AI actually works in clinical contexts.

Dr. John Torous (@John_Torous): Harvard psychiatrist researching digital mental health, including smartphone apps and AI. Publishes extensively on evidence base for digital mental health tools. Practical clinical focus.

NHS Digital and NHSX Leadership: Following official NHS digital health accounts provides policy updates, implementation guidance, and strategic direction.

Following 5-10 relevant thought leaders provides curated information flow without overwhelming your social media feeds. Mix clinical and technical perspectives for balanced understanding.

Conferences and Events:

DigitalHealth.London hosts regular events, webinars, and an annual major conference focused on health technology innovation in London and beyond.

Health 2.0 Europe: Annual conference bringing together healthcare organizations, innovators, and investors. More commercial than clinical but provides exposure to emerging technologies before they reach mainstream.

RCN Congress: Royal College of Nursing's annual conference increasingly includes digital health content. Nursing-specific perspective and networking opportunities.

NHS Expo: Annual event showcasing NHS innovations including AI implementations. Good for seeing real-world applications rather than just pilot projects.

Attending one major conference annually provides immersive learning and networking worth the time investment. Virtual attendance options increasingly available for those unable to travel.

14.5 The AI Ready Nurse

Throughout this textbook, we've explored AI's potential to transform mental health nursing and the substantial challenges that accompany that transformation. You've learned about specific technologies, ethical concerns, practical implementation, legal responsibilities, and professional evolution. But the deeper message has been about a mindset—approaching AI not with fear or uncritical enthusiasm, but with informed, critical engagement.

The AI-ready nurse isn't primarily defined by technical skills—though basic digital literacy helps. The AI-ready nurse is characterized by:

Critical thinking: Evaluating AI claims skeptically, demanding evidence, recognizing both potential and limitations, questioning whose interests technology serves.

Ethical commitment: Centering patient welfare, advocating for equitable AI that doesn't amplify inequalities, maintaining therapeutic relationships despite technological mediation, protecting privacy and autonomy.

Adaptive capacity: Willingness to learn continuously, experiment thoughtfully, acknowledge uncertainty, and adjust approaches based on evidence rather than defending initial positions.

Professional courage: Speaking up when AI implementations harm patients, challenging algorithms that don't serve clinical needs, advocating for nurse involvement in technology development, and maintaining clinical judgment even when algorithms recommend otherwise.

Collaborative orientation: Building networks, sharing knowledge, learning from colleagues' experiences, contributing to collective understanding rather than hoarding expertise.

These capacities matter more than knowing how any particular AI tool works. Technologies change; fundamental professional values and critical thinking abilities endure (Topol, 2019).

AI-ready nursing is patient advocacy in technological context. When algorithms produce biased recommendations, you speak up. When technologies are implemented primarily for institutional efficiency at patient expense, you challenge those decisions. When vendors make exaggerated claims, you demand evidence. When patients are confused or concerned about AI involvement in their care, you provide honest, informed explanations and respect their autonomy.

This advocacy role is deeply traditional nursing work applied to new circumstances. You've always advocated for patients against systems that disadvantaged them, insisted on evidence-based practice, maintained therapeutic relationships under challenging conditions, and adapted to changing healthcare environments. AI changes the specific challenges; it doesn't change your fundamental professional responsibilities.

The future of mental health nursing isn't predetermined. Technology companies, policymakers, healthcare administrators, and researchers are making choices now that will shape practice for decades. Nurses can influence those choices or be sidelined while others decide your profession's future. But influence requires engagement—learning about AI deeply enough to recognize good from bad implementations, building collective power through networks, developing expertise that makes you valuable to decision-makers, and refusing to accept technology that harms the people you're committed to serving.

This textbook has provided foundation. The next steps are yours. Pick one thing from Chapter 13.0's roadmap and do it this week. Join one professional network. Read one journal article about AI in mental health. Talk to one colleague about their digital health experiences. Each small action builds capacity and momentum.

The mental health nurses who thrive in an AI-augmented future won't be the ones who know the most about algorithms or use the most apps. They'll be the ones who maintain their core identity—as therapeutic, empathetic, critically-thinking advocates for vulnerable people—while thoughtfully integrating technology that genuinely serves patients. That's who you can be. That's who nursing needs you to be.

Appendices

Appendix A: Glossary of Key Terms

Algorithm: A set of rules or instructions that a computer follows to solve a problem or complete a task. In healthcare AI, algorithms analyze data to make predictions or recommendations.

Artificial Intelligence (AI): Computer systems that can perform tasks normally requiring human intelligence, such as pattern recognition, decision-making, and natural language understanding.

Chatbot: A computer program designed to simulate conversation with human users, often used for providing information or basic support in mental health applications.

Clinical Decision Support System (CDSS): Technology that provides healthcare professionals with knowledge and patient-specific information to inform clinical decisions.

Deep Learning: A type of machine learning using artificial neural networks with multiple layers. Particularly effective for complex pattern recognition tasks like analyzing medical images or speech.

Digital Phenotyping: Passive collection of behavioral data from smartphones and wearable devices to understand mental health status and changes over time.

Digital Therapeutics (DTx): Evidence-based therapeutic interventions delivered through software programs to prevent, manage, or treat medical conditions. Must demonstrate clinical effectiveness.

Machine Learning (ML): A subset of AI where systems learn from data and improve performance without being explicitly programmed for every scenario.

Natural Language Processing (NLP): AI technology that enables computers to understand, interpret, and generate human language. Used in chatbots and documentation analysis.

Predictive Analytics: Use of data, statistical algorithms, and machine learning to identify likelihood of future outcomes based on historical data.

Training Data: The dataset used to teach an AI algorithm to recognize patterns and make predictions. Quality and representativeness of training data critically affect algorithm performance.

Appendix B: AI Ethics Checklist

Use this checklist when evaluating AI tools for clinical use:

Patient Benefit and Safety

- [ ] Clear evidence that the tool improves patient outcomes or experience
- [ ] Benefits outweigh risks for the intended patient population
- [ ] Safety testing completed and documented
- [ ] Adverse events monitoring system in place
- [ ] Human oversight maintained for all clinical decisions

Informed Consent and Autonomy

- [ ] Patients informed about AI involvement in their care
- [ ] Clear explanation of how the tool works provided to patients
- [ ] Patients can opt out without penalty
- [ ] Consent process documented appropriately
- [ ] Patient preferences and values incorporated into AI-assisted decisions

Privacy and Data Protection

- [ ] Complies with GDPR and UK data protection law
- [ ] Data minimization principle followed (only necessary data collected)
- [ ] Secure data storage and transmission
- [ ] Clear data retention and deletion policies
- [ ] Patients understand how their data will be used

Fairness and Equity

- [ ] Training data includes diverse populations

- [ ] Algorithm tested for bias across demographic groups
- [ ] Performance disparities identified and addressed
- [ ] Tool accessible to patients with disabilities
- [ ] Doesn't systematically disadvantage marginalized groups

Transparency and Explainability

- [ ] Clinical reasoning behind AI recommendations understandable
- [ ] Limitations of the tool clearly stated
- [ ] Sources of training data disclosed
- [ ] Conflicts of interest declared
- [ ] Regular performance monitoring and reporting

Professional Accountability

- [ ] Clear roles and responsibilities for AI oversight
- [ ] Clinicians adequately trained to use the tool
- [ ] Documentation standards established
- [ ] Clinical judgment takes precedence over algorithmic recommendations
- [ ] Incident reporting processes for AI-related problems

Organizational Governance

- [ ] Information governance approval obtained
- [ ] Clinical governance oversight in place
- [ ] Evaluation plan established
- [ ] Resources allocated for proper implementation
- [ ] Mechanisms for discontinuing tool if harmful

Appendix C: Sample Patient Information Sheet

Using [AI Tool Name] in Your Mental Health Care

What is [Tool Name]? [Tool Name] is a digital program that [brief description of what it does—e.g., helps you track your mood and symptoms, provides therapeutic exercises, assesses your risk of crisis, etc.]. It uses artificial intelligence, which means it analyzes patterns in data to provide personalized recommendations or support.

How will it be used in my care? Your mental health nurse will [specific description—e.g., review your mood tracking data during appointments, use risk scores to help decide how frequently you need appointments, supplement face-to-face therapy with app-based exercises, etc.]. The tool provides information that helps your nurse make better decisions about your care, but your nurse remains responsible for all clinical decisions.

What information does it collect? [Specific data collected—e.g., your mood ratings, sleep patterns, activity levels, responses to questionnaires, smartphone usage patterns, etc.]. The information you enter or that is collected automatically stays confidential and is stored securely according to NHS data protection standards.

Do I have to use it? No. Using [Tool Name] is voluntary. You can decline without it affecting your access to mental health services. You can also stop using it at any time if you change your mind.

What are the benefits? [Specific benefits—e.g., your nurse will have better information about how you're doing between appointments, you'll have 24/7 access to support strategies, early warning signs of crisis can be detected sooner, etc.].

What are the risks? [Specific risks—e.g., the app might not always work properly, you might find tracking your mood increases your anxiety, the AI might miss warning signs that a human would notice, your data could potentially be accessed by unauthorized people if security is breached, etc.].

What if I have technical problems? Contact [specific support resource—your nurse, IT helpdesk, vendor support line, etc.]. [Include contact information].

What if I have concerns about my care? Speak with your mental health nurse first. If you're not satisfied, you can [escalation pathway—speak with team manager, contact PALS, formal complaints process, etc.].

Where can I learn more? [Links to additional information about the specific tool, general information about AI in healthcare, patient advocacy resources, etc.].

Appendix D: AI Tool Evaluation Template

Basic Information

- Tool name:
- Developer/vendor:
- Intended use:
- Target patient population:
- Cost:

Evidence Base

- Peer-reviewed research: (list studies)
- NICE guidance:
- Regulatory approval:
- Evidence quality rating:

Technical Specifications

- Platform (iOS, Android, web):
- Technical requirements:
- Integration with existing systems:
- Data storage location:
- Security features:

Clinical Utility

- Problem addressed:
- Expected benefits:
- Time investment required:
- Patient engagement factors:
- Clinician usability:

Equity and Bias

- Training data diversity:

- Performance across demographic groups:
- Accessibility features:
- Language options:
- Cultural appropriateness:

Governance

- Privacy policy adequacy:
- Data ownership clarity:
- Information governance compliance:
- Professional indemnity implications:
- Organizational approval status:

User Experience

- Patient feedback:
- Clinician feedback:
- Ease of use:
- Technical reliability:
- Support quality:

Overall Assessment

- Strengths:
- Limitations:
- Recommendation: (adopt / pilot / decline)
- Conditions for use:

Appendix E: Evidence-Based Digital Therapeutics

Condition	Tool	Evidence Level	NICE Status	Notes
Depression (mild-moderate)	SilverCloud	RCT evidence	Approved	Therapist-supported or self-directed CBT
Anxiety (various)	SilverCloud	RCT evidence	Approved	Multiple programs for different anxiety types
Insomnia	Sleepio	RCT evidence	Approved	6-week automated CBT for insomnia
PTSD	EMDR Therapy (app)	Preliminary evidence	Not reviewed	Supports EMDR between therapy sessions
Generalized support	Wysa	Preliminary evidence	In NHS Apps Library	AI chatbot, 24/7 availability
Substance use	WEconnect	Preliminary evidence	In NHS Apps Library	Recovery support and relapse prevention

Note: This table provides examples only, not comprehensive recommendations. Verify current evidence and regulatory status before clinical use. Tool availability and approval status change frequently.

Appendix F: Key Research Papers

Essential Reading for Mental Health Nurses Working with AI:

Torous, J., et al. (2020). The growing field of digital psychiatry: Current evidence and the future of apps, social media, chatbots, and virtual reality. *World Psychiatry*, 20(3), 318-335. *Comprehensive review of digital mental health technologies including AI applications.*

Obermeyer, Z., et al. (2019). Dissecting racial bias in an algorithm used to manage the health of populations. *Science*, 366(6464), 447-453. *Landmark study demonstrating algorithmic bias in healthcare and its mechanisms.*

Topol, E. J. (2019). High-performance medicine: The convergence of human and artificial intelligence. *Nature Medicine*, 25(1), 44-56. *Examines how AI can enhance rather than replace human clinicians.*

Char, D. S., et al. (2018). Implementing machine learning in health care—addressing ethical challenges. *New England Journal of Medicine*, 378(11), 981-983. *Overview of ethical issues in healthcare AI implementation.*

Graham, S., et al. (2019). Artificial intelligence for mental health and mental illnesses: An overview. *Current Psychiatry Reports*, 21(11), 116. *Comprehensive review of AI applications specific to mental health.*

Reference

- **Abdullah, S., Matthews, M., Murnane, E. L., Gay, G., & Choudhury, T.** (2014). Towards circadian computing: "Early to bed and early to rise" makes some of us unhealthy and sleep deprived. *Proceedings of the ACM International Joint Conference on Pervasive and Ubiquitous Computing*, 673–684.
- **Albert, P. R.** (2015). Why is depression more prevalent in women? *Journal of Psychiatry & Neuroscience*, 40(4), 219–221.
- **Andrews, G., Basu, A., Cuijpers, P., Craske, M. G., McEvoy, P., English, C. L., & Newby, J. M.** (2018). Computer therapy for the anxiety and depression disorders is effective, acceptable and practical health care: An updated meta-analysis. *Journal of Anxiety Disorders*, 55, 70–78.
- **Batal, H., Tench, J., McMillan, S., Adams, J., & Mehler, P. S.** (2001). Predicting patient visits to an urgent care clinic using calendar variables. *Academic Emergency Medicine*, 8(1), 48–53.
- **Bates, D. W., Saria, S., Ohno-Machado, L., Shah, A., & Escobar, G.** (2014). Big data in health care: Using analytics to identify and manage high-risk and high-cost patients. *Health Affairs*, 33(7), 1123–1131.
- **Beiwinkel, T., Kindermann, S., Maier, A., Kerl, C., Moock, J., Barbian, G., & Rössler, W.** (2016). Using smartphones to monitor bipolar disorder symptoms: A pilot study. *JMIR Mental Health*, 3(1), e2.
- **Belsher, B. E., Smolenski, D. J., Pruitt, L. D., Bush, N. E., Beech, E. H., Workman, D. E., … & Skopp, N. A.** (2019). Prediction models for suicide attempts and deaths: A systematic review and simulation. *JAMA Psychiatry*, 76(6), 642–651.
- **Benjamin, R.** (2019). *Race after technology: Abolitionist tools for the new Jim Code.* Polity Press.

- **Berger, T., Hämmerli, K., Gubser, N., Andersson, G., & Caspar, F.** (2011). Internet-based treatment of depression: A randomized controlled trial comparing guided with unguided self-help. *Cognitive Behaviour Therapy*, 40(4), 251–266.
- **Birchwood, M., Todd, P., & Jackson, C.** (2013). Early intervention in psychosis: The critical period hypothesis. *International Clinical Psychopharmacology*, 28(4), 184–187.
- **Bouwmans, M. E. J., Oude Oosterik, N. A. M., Bos, E. H., de Groot, I. W., Oldehinkel, A. J., & de Jonge, P.** (2018). The temporal order of changes in physical activity and subjective sleep in depressed versus nondepressed individuals: Findings from the MOOVD Study. *Behavioral Sleep Medicine*, 16(2), 154–168.
- **Buolamwini, J., & Gebru, T.** (2018). Gender shades: Intersectional accuracy disparities in commercial gender classification. *Proceedings of Machine Learning Research*, 81, 1–15.
- **Cabitza, F., Rasoini, R., & Gensini, G. F.** (2017). Unintended consequences of machine learning in medicine. *JAMA*, 318(6), 517–518.
- **Canzian, L., & Musolesi, M.** (2015). Trajectories of depression: Unobtrusive monitoring of depressive states by smartphone mobility traces. *Proceedings of the ACM International Joint Conference on Pervasive and Ubiquitous Computing*, 1293–1304.
- **Car, J., Gurol-Urganci, I., de Jongh, T., Vodopivec-Jamsek, V., & Atun, R.** (2012). Mobile phone messaging reminders for attendance at healthcare appointments. *Cochrane Database of Systematic Reviews*, 7, CD007458.
- **Char, D. S., Shah, N. H., & Magnus, D.** (2018). Implementing machine learning in health care—addressing ethical challenges. *New England Journal of Medicine*, 378(11), 981–983.
- **Chen, I. Y., Pierson, E., Rose, S., Joshi, S., Ferryman, K., & Ghassemi, M.** (2021). Ethical machine learning in healthcare. *Annual Review of Biomedical Data Science*, 4, 123–144.

- **Cheng, L. F., Dumitrascu, B., Zhang, M., Chivers, C., Draugelis, M., Li, K., & Engelhardt, B. E.** (2021). Sparse multi-output Gaussian processes for medical time series prediction. *BMC Medical Informatics and Decision Making*, 21(1), 1–23.
- **Chatterjee, H. J., Camic, P. M., Lockyer, B., & Thomson, L. J.** (2018). Non-clinical community interventions: A systematised review of social prescribing schemes. *Arts & Health*, 10(2), 97–123.
- **Coppersmith, G., Leary, R., Crutchley, P., & Fine, A.** (2018). Natural language processing of social media as screening for suicide risk. *Biomedical Informatics Insights*, 10, 1178222618792860.
- **Corcoran, C. M., Carrillo, F., Fernández-Slezak, D., Bedi, G., Klim, C., Javitt, D. C., … & Cecchi, G. A.** (2018). Prediction of psychosis across protocols and risk cohorts using automated language analysis. *World Psychiatry*, 17(1), 67–75.
- **Cummins, N., Scherer, S., Krajewski, J., Schnieder, S., Epps, J., & Quatieri, T. F.** (2015). A review of depression and suicide risk assessment using speech analysis. *Speech Communication*, 71, 10–49.
- **Digital Therapeutics Alliance.** (2021). What are digital therapeutics?
- **Erbe, D., Eichert, H. C., Riper, H., & Ebert, D. D.** (2017). Blending face-to-face and internet-based interventions for adults with mental disorders: Systematic review. *Journal of Medical Internet Research*, 19(9), e306.
- **Espie, C. A., Emsley, R., Kyle, S. D., Gordon, C., Drake, C. L., Siriwardena, A. N., … & Luik, A. I.** (2019). Effect of digital CBT-I on health, psychological well-being, and sleep-related quality of life: A randomized clinical trial. *JAMA Psychiatry*, 76(1), 21–30.
- **Eysenbach, G.** (2005). The law of attrition. *Journal of Medical Internet Research*, 7(1), e11.
- **Firth, J., Torous, J., Nicholas, J., Carney, R., Pratap, A., Rosenbaum, S., & Sarris, J.** (2017). The efficacy of smartphone-based mental health interventions for depressive

symptoms: Meta-analysis of RCTs. *World Psychiatry*, 16(3), 287–298.

- **Flett, J. A., Hayne, H., Riordan, B. C., Thompson, L. M., & Conner, T. S.** (2019). Mobile mindfulness meditation: A randomized controlled trial of two popular apps. *Mindfulness*, 10(5), 863–876.
- **Freeman, D., Reeve, S., Robinson, A., Ehlers, A., Clark, D., Spanlang, B., & Slater, M.** (2017). Virtual reality in the assessment, understanding, and treatment of mental health disorders. *Psychological Medicine*, 47(14), 2393–2400.
- **Furber, G., Crago, A., Meehan, K., Sheppard, T. D., Hooper, J., Hoeben, P., & Hoiles, K.** (2020). How adolescents use SMS for suicide prevention and the development of an SMS suicide prevention message. *Australasian Psychiatry*, 28(3), 244–248.
- **Fusar-Poli, P., McGorry, P. D., & Kane, J. M.** (2017). Improving outcomes of first-episode psychosis: An overview. *World Psychiatry*, 16(3), 251–265.
- **General Medical Council.** (2020). *Decision making and consent.*
- **Gianfrancesco, M. A., Tamang, S., Yazdany, J., & Schmajuk, G.** (2018). Potential biases in machine learning algorithms using EHR data. *JAMA Internal Medicine*, 178(11), 1544–1547.
- **Graham, S., Depp, C., Lee, E. E., Nebeker, C., Tu, X., Kim, H.-C., & Jeste, D. V.** (2019). Artificial intelligence for mental health and mental illnesses: An overview. *Current Psychiatry Reports*, 21(11), 116.
- **Greenhalgh, T., Wherton, J., Papoutsi, C., Lynch, J., Hughes, G., A'Court, C., … & Shaw, S.** (2017). Beyond adoption: The NASSS framework. *Journal of Medical Internet Research*, 19(11), e367.
- **Halvorsrud, K., Nazroo, J., Otis, M., Hajdukova, E. B., & Bhui, K.** (2019). Ethnic inequalities in diagnosis of severe mental illness in England: Systematic review and meta-analyses. *Social Psychiatry and Psychiatric Epidemiology*, 54(11), 1311–1323.

- **Hammana, I., Lepanto, L., Poder, T., Bellemare, C., & Ly, M. S.** (2015). Speech recognition in the radiology department: A systematic review. *Health Information Management Journal*, 44(2), 4–10.
- **Harvey, A. G.** (2008). Sleep and circadian rhythms in bipolar disorder: Seeking synchrony, harmony, and regulation. *American Journal of Psychiatry*, 165(7), 820–829.
- **Hirschberg, J., & Manning, C. D.** (2015). Advances in natural language processing. *Science*, 349(6245), 261–266.
- **Huberty, J., Green, J., Puzia, M. E., Larkey, L., Laird, B., Vranceanu, A. M., … & Vlisides-Henry, R.** (2021). Testing a mindfulness meditation mobile app for sleep-related symptoms: RCT. *PLOS ONE*, 16(1), e0244717.
- **Huckvale, K., Venkatesh, S., & Christensen, H.** (2019). Toward clinical digital phenotyping: Purpose, quality, and safety. *NPJ Digital Medicine*, 2, 88.
- **Huckvale, K., Torous, J., & Larsen, M. E.** (2019). Assessment of data sharing and privacy practices of apps for depression and smoking cessation. *JAMA Network Open*, 2(4), e192542.
- **ICO – Information Commissioner's Office.** (2017). Royal Free–Google DeepMind trial failed to comply with data protection law.
- **ICO – Information Commissioner's Office.** (2018). *Guide to the General Data Protection Regulation (GDPR).*
- **Inkster, B., Sarda, S., & Subramanian, V.** (2018). An empathy-driven conversational AI agent (Wysa) for digital mental well-being: Real-world mixed-methods evaluation. *JMIR mHealth and uHealth*, 6(11), e12106.
- **Kasparov, G.** (2017). *Deep thinking: Where machine intelligence ends and human creativity begins.* PublicAffairs.
- **Karyotaki, E., Riper, H., Twisk, J., Hoogendoorn, A., Kleiboer, A., Mira, A., … & Cuijpers, P.** (2017). Efficacy of self-guided internet-based CBT for depressive symptoms: IPD meta-analysis. *JAMA Psychiatry*, 74(4), 351–359.
- **Kirmayer, L. J., Fung, K., Rousseau, C., Lo, H. T., Menzies, P., Guzder, J., … & McKenzie, K.** (2021).

Guidelines for training in cultural psychiatry. *Canadian Journal of Psychiatry*, 66(2), 195–246.

- **Koutsouleris, N., Kahn, R. S., Chekroud, A. M., Leucht, S., Falkai, P., Wobrock, T., … & Hasan, A.** (2016). Multisite prediction of 4- and 52-week outcomes in first-episode psychosis: Machine learning approach. *The Lancet Psychiatry*, 3(10), 935–946.
- **Laranjo, L., Dunn, A. G., Tong, H. L., Kocaballi, A. B., Chen, J., Bashir, R., … & Coiera, E.** (2018). Conversational agents in healthcare: Systematic review. *Journal of the American Medical Informatics Association*, 25(9), 1248–1258.
- **LeCun, Y., Bengio, Y., & Hinton, G.** (2015). Deep learning. *Nature*, 521(7553), 436–444.
- **Lee, E. E., Depp, C., Graham, S., Nebeker, C., Tu, X., Kim, H.-C., & Jeste, D. V.** (2021). Artificial intelligence for mental healthcare: Clinical applications, barriers, facilitators. *Current Psychiatry Reports*, 23(11), 85.
- **Limbic.** (2023). Limbic Access: AI-powered mental health triage.
- **Lucas, G. M., Gratch, J., King, A., & Morency, L.-P.** (2014). It's only a computer: Virtual humans increase willingness to disclose. *Computers in Human Behavior*, 37, 94–100.
- **Marmot, M., Allen, J., Boyce, T., Goldblatt, P., & Morrison, J.** (2020). *Health equity in England: The Marmot review 10 years on.* Institute of Health Equity.
- **Martinez-Martin, N., Insel, T. R., Dagum, P., Greely, H. T., & Cho, M. K.** (2018). Data mining for health: Staking out the ethical territory of digital phenotyping. *NPJ Digital Medicine*, 1, 68.
- **Medicines and Healthcare products Regulatory Agency (MHRA).** (2023). Medical devices: Software applications (apps).
- **Medicines and Healthcare products Regulatory Agency (MHRA).** (2023). Software and AI as a medical device: Change programme.
- **Mitchell, T. M.** (1997). *Machine learning.* McGraw-Hill.

- **Mulholland, R., & Ulahannan, J. P.** (2020). Legal and ethical considerations for physicians in the digital age. *Postgraduate Medical Journal*, 96(1137), 428–431.
- **Musiat, P., Goldstone, P., & Tarrier, N.** (2014). Understanding the acceptability of e-mental health. *BMC Psychiatry*, 14, 109.
- **National Institute for Health and Care Excellence (NICE).** (2022). *Depression in adults: Treatment and management (NG222).*
- **NHS Digital.** (2023). Data security and protection toolkit.
- **NHS England.** (2023). Transformation Directorate: AI in health and care (AI Lab).
- **NHS England.** (2023). NHS digital mental health.
- **Nursing and Midwifery Council (NMC).** (2023). *The Code: Professional standards of practice and behaviour for nurses, midwives and nursing associates.*
- **Obermeyer, Z., Powers, B., Vogeli, C., & Mullainathan, S.** (2019). Dissecting racial bias in an algorithm used to manage the health of populations. *Science*, 366(6464), 447–453.
- **Onnela, J.-P., & Rauch, S. L.** (2016). Harnessing smartphone-based digital phenotyping to enhance behavioral and mental health. *Neuropsychopharmacology*, 41(7), 1691–1696.
- **Poissant, L., Pereira, J., Tamblyn, R., & Kawasumi, Y.** (2005). The impact of EHRs on time efficiency of physicians and nurses: Systematic review. *Journal of the American Medical Informatics Association*, 12(5), 505–516.
- **Powles, J., & Hodson, H.** (2017). Google DeepMind and healthcare in an age of algorithms. *Health and Technology*, 7(4), 351–367.
- **Price, W. N.** (2017). Regulating black-box medicine. *Michigan Law Review*, 116(3), 421–474.
- **Quiroz, J. C., Laranjo, L., Kocaballi, A. B., Berkovsky, S., Rezazadegan, D., & Coiera, E.** (2019). Challenges of developing a digital scribe to reduce clinical documentation burden. *NPJ Digital Medicine*, 2(1), 114.

- **Rajkomar, A., Hardt, M., Howell, M. D., Corrado, G., & Chin, M. H.** (2018). Ensuring fairness in machine learning to advance health equity. *Annals of Internal Medicine*, 169(12), 866–872.
- **Richards, D., Enrique, A., Eilert, N., Franklin, M., Palacios, J., Duffy, D., … & Timulak, L.** (2020). Digital interventions for depression and anxiety: Effectiveness and cost-effectiveness trial. *NPJ Digital Medicine*, 3, 85.
- **Richards, D., Timulak, L., O'Brien, E., Hayes, C., Vigano, N., Sharry, J., & Doherty, G.** (2015). An internet-delivered treatment as a low-intensity community intervention for depression: RCT. *Behaviour Research and Therapy*, 75, 20–31.
- **Rocher, L., Hendrickx, J. M., & de Montjoye, Y.-A.** (2019). Estimating the success of re-identifications in incomplete datasets using generative models. *Nature Communications*, 10, 3069.
- **Rosenbloom, S. T., Denny, J. C., Xu, H., Lorenzi, N., Stead, W. W., & Johnson, K. B.** (2011). Data from clinical notes: Tension between structure and flexible documentation. *Journal of the American Medical Informatics Association*, 18(2), 181–186.
- **Royal College of Nursing (RCN).** (2022). *Nursing workforce crisis: Employment survey 2022.*
- **Royal College of Nursing (RCN).** (2023). *Professional indemnity insurance: Information for RCN members.*
- **Rudin, C.** (2019). Stop explaining black box ML models for high-stakes decisions; use interpretable models instead. *Nature Machine Intelligence*, 1(5), 206–215.
- **Russell, S., & Norvig, P.** (2020). *Artificial intelligence: A modern approach* (4th ed.). Pearson.
- **Saeb, S., Lattie, E. G., Kording, K. P., & Mohr, D. C.** (2017). Mobile phone detection of semantic location and its relationship to depression and anxiety. *JMIR mHealth and uHealth*, 5(8), e112.
- **Saeb, S., Lattie, E. G., Schueller, S. M., Kording, K. P., & Mohr, D. C.** (2016). Mobile phone location sensor data and depressive symptom severity. *PeerJ*, 4, e2537.

- **Saeb, S., Zhang, M., Karr, C. J., Schueller, S. M., Corden, M. E., Kording, K. P., & Mohr, D. C.** (2015). Mobile phone sensor correlates of depressive symptom severity in daily life. *Journal of Medical Internet Research*, 17(7), e175.
- **Satinsky, E., Fuhr, D. C., Woodward, A., Sondorp, E., & Roberts, B.** (2019). Mental health care utilisation and access among refugees and asylum seekers in Europe: Systematic review. *Health Policy*, 123(9), 851–863.
- **Semigran, H. L., Linder, J. A., Gidengil, C., & Mehrotra, A.** (2015). Evaluation of symptom checkers for self-diagnosis and triage: Audit study. *BMJ*, 351, h3480.
- **Seifert, A., Cotten, S. R., & Xie, B.** (2021). A double burden of exclusion? Digital and social exclusion of older adults in times of COVID-19. *Journals of Gerontology: Series B*, 76(3), e99–e103.
- **Shaw, J., Rudzicz, F., Jamieson, T., & Goldfarb, A.** (2019). Artificial intelligence and the implementation challenge. *Journal of Medical Internet Research*, 21(7), e13659.
- **Topol, E. J.** (2019). High-performance medicine: The convergence of human and artificial intelligence. *Nature Medicine*, 25(1), 44–56.
- **Torous, J., Bucci, S., Bell, I. H., Kessing, L. V., Faurholt-Jepsen, M., Whelan, P., … & Firth, J.** (2020). The growing field of digital psychiatry: Apps, social media, chatbots, and virtual reality. *World Psychiatry*, 20(3), 318–335.
- **Torous, J., Kiang, M. V., Lorme, J., & Onnela, J.-P.** (2016). New tools for new research in psychiatry: A scalable platform for data-driven smartphone research. *JMIR Mental Health*, 3(2), e16.
- **Torous, J., & Roberts, L. W.** (2017). Needed innovation in digital health and smartphone applications for mental health: Transparency and trust. *JAMA Psychiatry*, 74(5), 437–438.
- **Tran, T., Luo, W., Phung, D., Harvey, R., Berk, M., Kennedy, R. L., & Venkatesh, S.** (2014). EMR-based risk

stratification better predicts suicide risk than clinician assessments. *BMC Psychiatry*, 14, 76.

- **Vayena, E., Salathé, M., Madoff, L. C., & Brownstein, J. S.** (2015). Ethical challenges of big data in public health. *PLOS Computational Biology*, 11(2), e1003904.
- **Wachter, S., Mittelstadt, B., & Floridi, L.** (2017). Why a "right to explanation" of automated decision-making does not exist in the GDPR. *International Data Privacy Law*, 7(2), 76–99.
- **Waller, G.** (2009). Evidence-based treatment and therapist drift. *Behaviour Research and Therapy*, 47(2), 119–127.
- **West, S. M., Whittaker, M., & Crawford, K.** (2019). *Discriminating systems: Gender, race, and power in AI.* AI Now Institute.
- **Yuste, R., Goering, S., Arcas, B. A. Y., Bi, G., Carmena, J. M., Carter, A., … & Wolpaw, J.** (2017). Four ethical priorities for neurotechnologies and AI. *Nature*, 551(7679), 159–163.
- **Zulueta, J., Piscitello, A., Rasic, M., Easter, R., Babu, P., Langenecker, S. A., … & Leow, A.** (2018). Predicting mood disturbance severity with mobile phone keystroke metadata: BiAffect study. *Journal of Medical Internet Research*, 20(7), e241.

www.ingramcontent.com/pod-product-compliance
Lightning Source LLC
LaVergne TN
LVHW052323200926
848481LV00002B/648
9781923646148